MELANY CAR

COMPULSIVE OVEREATING

KNOW HOW TO RECOVERY YOUR BODY, WHAT TO EAT AND RESCUE YOUR EMOTION!

CBT, EMDR, MUSIC THERAPY AND TIPS FOR HEALING YOUR MIND AND SOUL FROM BINGE, BULIMIA AND ANOREXIA DISORDERS!

COPYRIGHT

SOMMARIO

INTRODUCTION

Eating Disorders (DCA) include Anorexia, Nervous Bulimia, Not Otherwise Specified Eating Disorders (Partial Syndromes) and Binge Eating Disorders (Binge Eating Disorder).

The latter category, recently described in the Diagnostic and Statistical Manual of Mental Disorders of the American Psychiatric Association (DSM IV), has a status still to be defined.

Recent nosography, in particular the Diagnostic and Statistical Manual of Mental Disorders of the American Psychiatric Association, 4th edition, in the chapter dedicated to Eating Disorders includes Nervous Anorexia and Nervous Bulimia, the most common eating disorders and N.A.S. Eating Disorders (less specific or less typical). In the Appendix, for the new categories being studied, the Uncontrolled Eating Disorder (Compulsive) has been inserted instead. Among all these disorders the most common and therefore most studied are Anorexia and Bulimia.

ISTAT statistics (2000) report that out of a population of 4,600,000 young Italian women aged between 12 and 25, an estimated 138,000 cases of anorexia and 230,000 cases of bulimia are estimated. The first manifestation of Anorexia is recorded on average towards the

17 years old. STS-DCA experts have identified two peaks with respect to the frequency of onset age, one around the age of 14, the other at 18. Pre-pubertal anorexia are more rare, before the characteristic somatic changes of puberty and premenarcal occur. Bulimia is a syndrome of recent definition, therefore the epidemiological data are less.

Food Behaviour Disorders (EDCs) prevail especially in Western industrialized countries where thinness is a socially important and "desirable" value: they are victims of it.

45 % of girls between the ages of 15 and 35. This cultural model is disseminated through messages conveyed by magazines, films, television and advertising that lead back to the respect and kindness of a person to the "perfect physical shape". Western teenagers resort to the stereotype of women proposed by the world of fashion, in the continuous search for the approval of others. In today's society, the female figure is subject to demands that are often irreconcilable and contradictory, forcing her to be a

caring wife and mother, an attractive and well-groomed woman, and at the same time to compete intellectually and professionally with men. Excessive concern about physical forms, control of the act of eating, the thought of food, easily become obsessive behaviors that can conceal a deeper disease: this affects fundamentally young women who, while fighting against their bodies, fight desperately, in reality, even against the feeling of not being able to lead their own lives independently. To be thin, to maintain one's own weight for these people means to correspond to the ideal of thinness propagated by fashion (a standardized identity) and at the same time to deny the feminine characteristics (that is, welcoming, receptive) of the body, felt as little responding to the requirements of strength and effectiveness, which are so often required of the woman of today. The eating disorders also affect the male world, even if in a minority (5%), highlighting the evolution of a cultural context that increasingly reduces the differences between roles male and female. The female world is more susceptible to these diseases because it is subject to more frequent diets, which increase the likelihood of developing eating disorders. The relationship with food is relevant in the

3

formation of the identity of males and post-modern females, as it is related to both self-perception and interaction with the world. Approval is based on physical appearance and thinness. A physical aspect becomes more important than anything else and on it is based the self-assessment that the patient has of himself.

Nervous Anorexia, despite the interest it has had over the centuries (see for example the fasting of many saints), still remains today, in some respects, an interpretative enigma. The most striking aspect is the woman with a male/female ratio of 1:10 to 1:20; "this is the most unbalanced sex ratio of all psychiatric disorders". It is a pathology that affects mind and body, childhood and adult life and, therefore, is difficult to describe through the language of medicine and psychiatry, so as to be defined as "enigma". The term Anorexia derives from the negative prefix "a" and from the Greek verb "orego" which means to wish: the literal meaning therefore emphasizes a lack of desire more than a the willingness to refuse food. In anorexics there is an attitude of food rejection which does not, however, lead to a lack of appetite but is instead linked to the strong fear of fattening and the need to control food. "Not eating means purifying

4

oneself from the sense of guilt for the hatred that comes out of the relationship with the mother on whom one is tremendously dependent". Much information on anorexia comes to us from the medieval period, although most scholars wonder about the possibility of commensurate the current cases of frank anorexia nervosa to the strict practices of fasting in a cultural context steeped in mysticism such as the Middle Ages. The first description of a case that presents the clinical characteristics of the current Anorexia Nervosa dates back to the sixteenth century, by Simone Portio, Neapolitan philosopher, who refers to a young girl who was reduced to conditions of extreme thinness by spontaneous fasting. The first official clinical description is instead that of the English doctor Richard Morton, who in 1689 published his Treatise "Phthisiology: or a Treatise ori Consumption", in which he reported a syndrome of depletion of nervous origin, characterized by loss of global appetite, without fever or cough, or altered breathing, accompanied by amenorrhea, constipation, extreme slimming, incessant activity of the patient and a real rejection of any treatment. Morton assumed that the cause of the disease was to be found in the central nervous system (i.e. in the mind), stating that

5

everything had begun "for a multitude of cares and passions of her mind"(1689).

In the second half of the 19th century, doctors Charles Lasegue in France (1873) and William Gull in Great Britain (1874) published some works on cases of voluntary fasting, now recognizable as anorexia. The Bulimia, which etymologically means "ox hunger" (from the Greek bous=bue + limos=fame), appears rarely mentioned, before the seventies, in medical publications. Considered until the end of the last century and in the early twentieth century a component of the clinical picture of Anorexia, the Bulimia has now been recognized, in the DSM, as an entity in its own right. In 1979 Professor Gerald Russel claimed that Bulimia was a clinical variable of mental anorexia, later it was related to obesity, until it was described as an autonomous syndrome.

Bulimia became more known with the dissemination of data documenting the increase of overfeeding and voluntary emptying of the stomach in American university colleges.

To date, a low percentage of bulimic subjects require professional help because of the strong feelings of guilt and shame that accompany long periods of inadequate eating habits. This makes it difficult to research the incidence of Bulimia.

To date, the therapies most used for the treatment of DCA are Cognitive Behavioral Therapy (CBT) and Interpersonal Psychotherapy (IPT), which, although they have shown to be effective in the treatment of this disease, have some limitations, including the fact that they do not give particular and primary importance to the intervention on traumatic experiences, both in the onset and maintenance of DCA.

The Eye Movement Desensitization and Reprocessing (EMDR) therapy successfully tackles this limit; in fact, it goes beyond the purely behavioral point of view and allows to go deep into the mechanisms of onset of the disorder.

In line with this, the objective of this thesis is to analyze the role of trauma in the genesis and maintenance of Bulimia Nervosa, adopting as a theoretical model of reference the theory of adaptive information processing, typical of EMDR, and as a treatment model the EMDR therapy with its eight phases, designed to take charge of a pathology as complex as food.

.

CHAPTER 1:

BULIMIA NERVOSA AND ITS TRAUMATIC ORIGINS

NOSOGRAPHIC CLASSIFICATION OF THE NERVOUS BULIMIA

The term "bulimia" comes from the Greek "" and literally means "ox hunger". For many centuries this term has been used to indicate a symptom secondary to various forms of mental disorders and brain disorders and concerning an uncontrollable urge to eat large amounts of food.

Its meaning as a syndrome has only recently appeared; it was, in fact, since 1979 by the psychiatrist Gerald Russell that bulimia was understood as an autonomous nosographic entity. The author, publishing in the journal "Psychological Medicine" an article entitled "Bulimia Nervosa: an Ominous Variant of Anorexia Nervosa", defined it as a syndrome characterized by the morbid fear of fattening, uncontrollable crises of greed and dangerous behaviors of compensation aimed at avoiding weight gain.

Since then, this syndrome has appeared in the third edition of the statistical and diagnostic manual of mental disorders (DSM-III), under the name of Russell di Bulimia Nervosa, precisely to avoid terminological confusion with bulimia-symptom and to emphasize its close link with Anorexia Nervosa (De Giacomo et al., 2005).

CLASSIFICATION AND DIAGNOSIS ACCORDING TO DSM-5

The latest version of the Mental Disorder Diagnostic Manual, known as DSM-5, classifies Bulimia Nervosa within the "Nutrition and Nutrition Disorders" section, which also includes pica, rumination disorder, food intake avoidance/restriction disorder, anorexia nervosa (type with restrictions and type with binges/elimination pipelines), uncontrolled eating disorder, other specified nutrition or eating disorder, and unspecified nutrition or eating disorder.

All these diseases, although different from each other, are characterized by "a persistent eating disorder or dietary behavior that results in altered food consumption or absorption and that significantly affects physical health or psychosocial functioning.

Currently the diagnostic criteria for diagnosing bulimia nervosa are:

Recurrent episodes of binge eating. An episode of binge eating is characterized by both of the following aspects:

eating in a given period of time (e.g., a two-hour period) a significantly greater amount of food than most individuals would eat at the same time and in similar circumstances;

feeling of losing control during the episode (e.g. feeling of not being able to stop eating or control what and how much you are eating).

Recurrent and inappropriate compensatory conduct to prevent weight gain, such as self-induced vomiting, abuse of laxatives, diuretics or other medications, fasting or excessive physical activity.

Inappropriate binges and compensatory conduct both occur on average at least once a week for 3 months.

Levels of self-esteem are unduly influenced by body shape and weight.

The alteration does not occur exclusively during episodes of Anorexia Nervosa.

Compared to DSM-IV-TR, the minimum number of binges and inappropriate compensatory behaviors useful for diagnosis is reduced (from 2 to 1 per week for 3 months), the distinction between purgative and non-purgatory subtypes is abolished and, finally, the clinician is given the possibility to specify the level of severity of the disorder. In fact, with respect to the latter, the DSM-5 allows, based on the frequency of inappropriate compensatory conduct, to specify the current level of severity of the disorder, distinguishing between:

mild: an average of 1-3 episodes of inappropriate compensatory conduct per week;

moderate: an average of 4-7 episodes of inappropriate compensatory conduct per week;

severe: an average of 8-13 episodes of inappropriate compensatory conduct per week;

extreme: an average of 14 or more episodes of inappropriate compensatory conduct per week.

EPIDEMIOLOGICAL DATA

As far as epidemiological data are concerned, they are mainly derived from the diagnosis and it is important to underline in this sense that eating disorders (DCA) are often denied or hidden by those who suffer from them, which makes epidemiological studies difficult and expensive.

"Many studies use data from health services to assess the number of these disorders, but the results are usually underestimated, as not all patients go to a medical facility. In some cases it is a small minority.

Estimates of the prevalence of NL suggest that this disorder is slightly more frequent than Anorexia Nervosa (AN). In fact, a rapid sequence of changes in the relative frequency of the various forms of psychopathology of eating behaviour has been reported: in the 1960s, the most common clinical pictures were the restrictive anorexia, and in the following decades, the bulimic forms became increasingly frequent.

According to the studies conducted by Hoek H.W. and Van Hoeken D. (2003), the NL would have a prevalence rate of 1% in the case of women and 0.1% in the case of men, while the incidence would be equal to 12 per 100,000 people per year.

The National Comorbidity Survey Replication Study, whose data refer to surveys carried out on a large random sample representative of the US population, recorded a lifetime prevalence rate5 of 1.5% in the

13

case of women and 0.5% in the case of men. Although these studies were based on reliable data, they were carried out on the basis of the criteria of the DSM-IV-TR. To overcome this limit, two recent reviews have evaluated the epidemiology of DCA in the light of the new criteria of the DSM-5, reporting for the NL an annual incidence of 300 cases per 100,000 and a lifetime prevalence of 2%.

As far as the Italian situation is concerned, it is found that: the incidence of NL is at least 12 new cases per 100,000 people in one year among women and about 0.8 new cases per 100,000 people in one year among men; the point prevalence is between 0.5 and 1.8% among young women; the lifetime prevalence, in the general population over 18 years of age, is 1.5% among women and 0.5% among men. In women aged between 18 and 24 years, the rates for NL are much higher, about 4.5%. It is therefore clear that NL is more frequent in the female population than in the male population (Cuzzolaro, 2014). In the studies conducted on clinical populations, men make up 10-15% of the cases of NL 7 and, although this represents a minority, at the same time this percentage reflects an increase in cases, linked in part to a greater importance that our society gives to fitness and a greater use of health services by male subjects. With regard to the spread of NL in industrialized and non industrialized countries, the numerous epidemiological studies that have dealt with this topic have highlighted how the incidence of these diseases is greater in industrialized countries (Western Europe, United States, Canada, Australia, New Zealand, Japan, South Africa) and is strongly related to the economic development and values of Western culture.

DEVELOPMENT AND PROGRESS

The age of onset of the NL is placed with a greater incidence during the period of adolescence and young adult age, between 15 and 19 years.

Early onset forms, as well as late onset forms, following menopause, are rare. The development of the disorder may occur in relation to a severe dietary restriction to change body weight or as a result of emotional difficulties in dealing with stressful situations. Bulimic crises are usually triggered by the breaking of extreme dietary rules, dysphoric moods, subjectively stressful events and feelings of emptiness and loneliness. In most cases they are followed by compensatory practices (such as self-induced vomiting, improper use of laxatives and/or diuretics, excessive physical exercise and fasting) which, although on the one hand they help to keep weight within normal range, on the other hand they can have, together with malnutrition and excessive eating (particularly of fats and carbohydrates), a series of medical consequences.

The main medical complications that are found in subjects with BN are:
-on the skin, dryness of the skin, acne, alopecia (patchy hair loss), lanugo (fine hair), Russel's sign (callosity on the back of the hand caused by rubbing of the fingers against the dental arch), perioral irritations (inflammation on the lip contour due to regurgitated acid juices), petechiae on the face, conjunctival hemorrhages and/or subcutaneous emphysema (presence of air in the subcutaneous tissues);
-in the orogastrointestinal system, dental enamel erosion, dental caries, gingivitis, hypertrophy of the salivary glands, esophageal, gastric, pancreatic and gastro-intestinal problems;

-at an electrolytic level, a series of imbalances, such as hypopotassemia, leading to electrocardiographic abnormalities;

-at the cardiovascular level, sinus bradycardia (heart rate < 60 beats per minute), arterial hypotension (systolic pressure < 90 mmHg and/or diastolic pressure < 50mmHg), ventricular arrhythmias, mitral and tricuspid valve prolapse, electrocardiocadiographic abnormalities (such as lengthening of the QT tract);

-at the respiratory level, spontaneous pneumothorax (accumulation of air in the pleural cavity with consequent collapse of the lungs), emphysema (lung disease caused by deterioration of the alveoli that allow the exchange of respiratory gases between the blood and the atmosphere) and pneumonia from ingestion (caused by the entry of foreign substances into the bronchopulmonary tree);

-metabolic level, hypercholesterolemia and/or hyperinsulinemia; at the neuro-endocrine level, hypercortisolemia and increased secretion of dehydroepiandrosterone on the hypothalamus-pituitary surrene axis, secretion of the stimulating follicle hormone (FSH), of the leutenizing hormone (LH), of estrogens and progesterone on the hypothalamus-pituitary-gonadic axis, increase in growth hormone and hyperprolactinemia.

The course of the BN can be chronic or intermittent, with remission phases alternating with reappearance phases of binge eating. The rate of remission is about 27% one year after onset and over 70% after 10 years or more. Diagnostic cross-over from bulimia nervosa to anorexia nervosa occurs in a minority of cases (10-15%), while more frequent (up to 20%) is the shift to other eating disorders and binge-eating disorder.

About 23% of patients have a chronic course that persists throughout their lives, severely damaging interpersonal functioning and their school or work careers. This picture seems to be worse when associated with obesity, low self-esteem and personality disorders.

The mortality rate is high. According to DSM-5 it is about 2% per decade and is partly linked to the risk of suicide, which is high among patients suffering from BN. A recent study found a 26.9% proportion of people who attempted suicide among a sample of 566 women who suffered from BN at least once in their lifetime. This autolegive behaviour is closely related to a low level of education, diagnosis of childhood obesity, history of alcohol abuse by a family member (in particular, by a parent), presence of impulsive behaviour (i.e. substance abuse, kleptomania, compulsive shopping, autolegive behaviour), lack of self-awareness, sense of ineffectiveness, interpersonal difficulties, internalizing (as damage avoidance) and externalizing (as impulsiveness, anxiety and borderline personality disorder) personality traits, which could be the main responsible for the high frequency of this type of acts among subjects suffering from BN.

EATING DISORDER AND COMORBIDITY

The BN frequently manifests itself in comorbidity with another mental disorder, usually related to the sphere of mood disorders or anxiety disorders.

Compared to mood disorders, it has been observed that in individuals with BN there is an increased frequency of depressive symptoms (e.g., low self-esteem) and bipolar and depressive disorders. Literature reviews show that 50 to 70 % of people suffering from BN experience higher rates of depression during their lifetime than the general population. In many individuals, mood disorder begins at the same time as or following the development of NL, but there are also cases where it occurs earlier. Not infrequently, in fact, subjects identify it as the cause of bulimia itself.

Compared to anxiety disorders, it has emerged that there may be an increased frequency of anxiety symptoms or anxiety disorders.

In addition to depression and anxiety disorders, a comorbidity was observed between BN and substance use disorders (especially alcohol and stimulants). It was found that the lifetime prevalence of this disorder is at least 30% among individuals suffering from BN.

With regard to personality disorders and BN, a significant proportion of individuals show comorbidities with one or more personality disorders. There is, in fact, ample evidence of the prevalence of personality disorders (DP) among patients suffering from DCA. Among these, the most frequent are borderline personality disorder and avoidant personality disorder, followed by obsessive-compulsive, paranoid and dependent personality disorder.

FACTORS THAT DROWN IN EATING DISORDER

A sort of pendulum has oscillated in the search for the factors responsible for the NL, passing from organic to psychological and environmental factors. The various schools of thought, which have questioned the causes, have highlighted different factors, emphasizing each time strictly organic hypotheses (damage of the pituitary gland, injury of the hunger center, genetic disease) or more specifically psychological and relational (personality characteristics, family structure).

Today, the scientific community tends to propose multifactorial models for this disorder, which are based on a bio-psycho-social perspective and agrees that there is no single cause but a combination of factors that can interact differently and variously between them in favor of the appearance and perpetuation. In today's society, in fact, everyone is exposed to the excessive supply of food and, at the same time, to the constant presentation of images of lean bodies. Many people worry about what they eat and how much they eat, often undertaking unjustified diets to reduce dissatisfaction with their physical appearance. So why do only a few of these people get sick from serious eating disorders?

The multifactorial model, which sees the pathological event as the common final path of various possible pathogenetic processes, invites us to keep in mind a long series of factors and events, some of which play an important role with respect to a biological and psychological vulnerability to the disorder (predisposing factors), others in the transition from vulnerability to the actual disorder (precipitating factors) and, finally, others in the formation of a vicious circle that develops and maintains the disease.

PREDISPOSING FACTORS

According to some, there may be factors predisposing to all possible causes that can predispose and facilitate the onset of the problem. They can be divided into the following categories:

General risk factors

General risk factors are those non-modifiable conditions that increase the risk of developing an eating disorder; among these, the conditions that cause the greatest increase in risk are gender, female, and age, i.e. adolescence and early adulthood.

As far as women are concerned, the reasons why women are affected more than men are not fully known. According to a psychological and social hypothesis, the key factor is the different frequency between the two sexes in undertaking a diet: women, being more exposed to social pressures and basing their value on physical appearance, tend more frequently to put on a diet.

As far as the age of onset is concerned, the development of eating disorders in adolescence and early adulthood is likely to be favoured by the interaction of biological factors (e.g. hormonal variations, synapse remodelling and progressive myelination of nerve fibres) and environmental factors (e.g. stressful events, environmental challenges). In adolescence, in fact, we go through a complex process of separation / differentiation from parents, the identity is not yet well defined and there is a strong tendency to judge their value in terms of physical appearance, in addition to this, there are profound physical changes, especially in girls with an increase in body fat, which can promote a body away from the current aesthetic ideal and a decrease in the level of personal satisfaction. Finally, always in adolescence, there can be various stressful situations that can threaten the sense of self-control, and diet and weight loss, with the consequent assumption of prepubescent physical and psychological characteristics, can be a means to achieve a sense of self-control.

GENETIC RISK FACTORS

Genetic risk factors are the wide range of genetic variants that give an individual specific vulnerability to the development of a DCA. According to the study of endophenotypes, there are some hereditary characteristics (e.g. perfectionism and cognitive rigidity) for dietary diseases that seem to contribute to the predisposition to the disease and that seem to be present even in the absence of the disease itself. These endophenotypes have been found in healthy relatives of sick people with a higher frequency than the general population. Studies of epigenetics argue that early exposure to certain environmental situations (such as obesogenic environment, poor nutrition, early trauma or stress) may increase the susceptibility to develop an epigenetic eating disorder in adulthood. The environment, in fact, contributes to determine and modify the phenotype (observable characteristic) also through particular alterations of the genome, which do not involve profound changes in the DNA, but pass through chemical processes that affect the DNA itself and the histones. Epigenetic alterations have therefore been reported, linked to reduced dopaminergic activity in women with borderline personality disorder, bulimic symptoms and a history of physical and sexual abuse in childhood.

Transgenerational studies have shown that there is a higher risk of BN among relatives of patients with DCA than among relatives of healthy subjects. The data indicate that relatives of people with DCA have a risk of developing the disorder about ten times higher than those without; the genetic component in the family transmission of NL is therefore relevant. Studies on twins in the general population have shown a heritability ranging from 28% to 83% for NL, showing a higher concordance rate for monozygotic twins than for heterozygotic twins.

Still considering the role of genetic risk factors, some researches have shown, even if with heterogeneous results, a reduced functionality of the serotonergic, dopaminergic, noradrenergic system at cortical level and neuroendocrine modifications (ghrelin, leptin, cholecystokinin, neutrophic factor of central derivation, etc.) at peripheral level, which involve not only the alteration of the sense of hunger and satiety, but also the genesis and/or maintenance of binge eating. However, it is not yet well known whether these alterations should be considered a cause or a consequence (or both) of the eating disorder.

SOCIO-CULTURAL RISK FACTORS

The socio-cultural aspects are factors of primary importance in the development of the NL, which not by chance has been defined, a "cultural syndrome". In today's globalized society, the dominant aesthetic ideal, transversal to different social, economic and cultural contexts, imposes the value of the "lean body". This is accompanied by the stigmatization of obesity, which from a health problem ends up becoming a reprehensible condition to be ashamed of, an emblem of personal failure. In this idealization of thinness, the mass media seem to play an important role, which, in addition to emphasizing the messages on the desirability of a thin body, encourage the use of the most varied and often unrealistic strategies to pursue the ideal of beauty; what follows is the formation of a disturbed body image.

The feeling of inadequacy caused by the discrepancy between the current physical appearance and the models proposed by the mass media can lead to restrictive diets (a powerful correlatum of the NL) and to pursue the ideal of thinness as a form of the symptom through which to express one's malaise in an attempt to seek relief. In addition to this, an important role in everyday life and, more than any other, in that of young people is played by the Internet. In the web there are almost three hundred thousand sites that exalt the anorexic female model, making anorexia and bulimia pass for "fashion"; among these noteworthy are "pro-anorexia", "pro-axa" and "anorexic nation", which represent a powerful risk factor for the development of the NL (Balbo, 2017). They represent both predisposing factors and precipitating and perpetuating factors, given their negative and, at the same time, reinforcing effects on self-esteem (Cuzzolaro, 2014).

INDIVIDUAL RISK FACTORS

The presence of overweight in childhood and preadolescence is a risk factor for the development of NL. Some studies have, in fact, shown that the predisposition to obesity, in a context that emphasizes the value of thinness, can promote body dissatisfaction, the possibility of being exposed to criticism and teasing, excessive concern for the weight and shape of the body and the adoption of inappropriate behaviors for weight reduction.

On a strictly psychological level, among the characteristics identified as possible factors predisposing to the development of the NL there are: borderline personality traits, perfectionism, exasperated expectations, great difficulties in the process of separation-identification, low self-esteem, disordered sexuality, dependence on the consent and admiration of others, fixation on childhood and childhood forms of dependence and control, pathological narcissism, poor control of impulses, intolerance of frustration, tendency to sudden changes in mood. Individual risk factors may also include lack of self-awareness. In fact, the inability to identify and express one's own internal states can lead the individual to feel confused and not to consider one's own feelings reliable, secondarily developing pathological eating behaviours in order to compensate for this deficit.

FAMILY RISK FACTORS

Some familiar factors that may play a risk role in the onset of the NL have been reported. In the past, many theories have wrongly placed the family, particularly the mother, in the dock, establishing linear causal correlations between the behavior of parents and the onset of the disorder in children. The result was to generate blame and guilt.

Today, the most accredited opinion is that most of the problems observed in families with a child with an eating disorder are the consequence and not the cause of the disorder itself. However, this should not lead to a lack of awareness of the influence that the family can have on the genesis of the disorder; food is, in fact, one of the main vehicles of relations between mother and child. Food interaction is one of the first and main areas in which communication takes place and this non-verbal transaction remains a foundation of neurophysiological and intrapsychological patterns that will organize the child's future experiences.

Among the traits present in family members, prior to the onset of an eating disorder, we can identify elements of anxiety, compulsiveness and disturbed nutrition (impulse to thinness, control of eating behavior, anorexia and bulimia). An insecure, depressed, anxious caregiver or one with dysfunctional eating habits in front of a crying child may find in the provision of food an easy way to reward or calm him down, resolving his anxiety, but not learning to recognize the real needs of the child, who will accept the food as a caregiver. The style of attachment that most frequently appears to be present in patients with BN is the insecure ambivalent/resistant and/or disorganized style of attachment. This underlines how a psychological vulnerability of the caregiver constitutes a predictive variable of a future eating disorder and of difficulties in the emotional sphere of the child. Dysfunctional socioaffective experiences17 can, in fact, interfere with the development of self-regulatory abilities, with initiatives of autonomy, with feelings of trust, self-efficacy of the child (self-reliance) and with the drive to master situations (mastery), generating a low nuclear self-esteem which, together with other factors, may constitute a risk factor for the onset of a food disorder.

In addition to this, the construction of the body image and the consequent satisfaction-in dissatisfaction with one's physical appearance are also linked to the quality of the attachment relationship with both parents. For example, the father's reaction to the maturation of the daughter's body in adolescence can play an important role in the formation of the daughter's feelings towards her body.

PRECIPITATING FACTORS

The precipitating factors are those factors that increase the risk of developing the eating disorder and, among these, there are also those life events, to which the most vulnerable people give a disturbing meaning, intolerable to the point of triggering the disease. These events are no different from those reported for the onset of other psychiatric diseases and this highlights the importance of the predisposing factors in the choice of the symptom. Noteworthy triggers include:

PUBERTY

Empirical data show that puberty timing should be considered a relevant risk factor. This process generally begins between 8 and 13 years in girls and between 9 and 14 years in males, although there is no lack of significant individual differences with early or delayed starts compared to the average.

During puberty the female body is shaped by an increase in fat mass, curves in the region of the hips and belly and hair in different parts of the body. These changes are in sharp contrast to the canons imposed by Western society, which would like girls tall, thin, free of body fat and glabrous. It is, therefore, understandable that girls who have a high Body Mass Index (BMI) and a presence of fat mass are less satisfied with their body. Moreover, it is at this age that the appearance of the menarche, hormonal storms, secondary sexual characteristics, sexual desires, changes in one's gaze on oneself and on others and that of others on oneself occurs. All of this can only have repercussions on the lifestyle of girls and on the perception of their changing bodies.

A wide range of research has suggested that dissatisfaction with one's body and problems related to body image are also present in the male population: studies on the preadolescent and adolescent male population have shown that both underweight and overweight are associated with higher levels of body dissatisfaction and concern for their image. It follows that weight variation can become something painful and embarrassing for the most vulnerable; they, in fact, begin to experience an event physiologically related to age as a reason for shame in the culture of thinness. These subjects, in a condition of emotional turbulence, anxiety, impulsiveness, underestimation of risks, can react with an obsessive concentration on the body, weight and / or diet, in order to regain a feeling of value and control over the metamorphosis taking place.

Relationship with peers and negative criticism of one's physical appearance

In adolescence, family relationships tend to lose importance, while those with peers are gaining more and more importance, dissatisfaction with the image of the body due to comparisons, devaluations and derisions.

CHANGES

Changes, such as school changes or family changes, can alter the psychological, biological and social balance of some people, creating strong stress. Although stress is an inevitable and even functional component in everyone's life, when it exceeds it, it can become dysfunctional and compromise the subject's ability to adapt, causing a lack of perceived self-efficacy, low self-esteem and a sense of impotence. To cope with this sense of cognitive, physical and emotional overwhelming, some individuals, particularly women, may run the risk of developing an eating disorder. Excessive control over diet, weight and body shape can, in fact, be read as a dysfunctional way of coping with unpredictable events and threats from the surrounding environment.

MOURNING FOR A LOVED AND SIGNIFICANT PERSON

A great deal of research has shown that the loss of a loved one can be followed, in a not inconsiderable number of people, by a clinically significant discomfort both physically and mentally. When a loved one dies, the individual no longer perceives his or her world as a stable and safe place, his or her daily habits are upset and he or she feels an explosion of emotions that cannot be processed. This separation can be experienced as an unbridgeable void and this can lead the most vulnerable to resort to food and/or excessive control over their bodies as a way of managing and expressing suffering. The reaction to mourning can, in fact, determine a low self-esteem, a sense of emptiness, as well as a loss of control.

TRAUMA AND SEXUAL ABUSE

In the DCA, as in many other psychiatric pathologies, traumatic experiences of emotional deprivation and sexual abuse in childhood and adolescence may be at stake as predisposing or precipitating factors.

34

Trauma, in fact, given its particularly painful emotional experience, can have a disorganizing effect on the psychobiological system of the person, becoming a risk factor for the NL.

THE DIET

Dieting, or "dieting", is an important risk factor for the development of eating disorders in normal-weight adolescents. In a sample of fifteen-year-old London students, those on a diet, compared to controls, had an eight-fold higher risk of developing an eating disorder in the following year. Similar results were observed in a study of Australian adolescents in whom dietary subjects, compared to non-diet subjects, had an eighteen-fold higher risk of developing a DCA in the following six months.

Adolescence is, in fact, a period of strong development from the physical point of view and the need to adhere to the cultural models of beauty imposed by Western society can lead to inappropriate eating habits, including poorly managed or self-imposed diets, which today represent an increasingly widespread practice, which do not take into account the possible risk factors for the person. These diets, in fact, if not adapted to the energy needs of age, can: induce chronic hunger, give rise to episodes of uncontrolled eating, when cognitive control is lacking, and generate, because of the social reinforcements associated with losing weight and the perception of control that is associated with it, dangerous spirals, such as the cycle restriction-buffate-restriction that is the hallmark of the NL.

THE REPETITION OF CONFIRMATIONS FOR DCAS

Why do the DCAs keep going? What are the perpetuating factors that make them continue as wrong behaviours? These are all those behaviours and factors that confirm and reinforce the dysfunctional behaviour of the subject:

Excessive assessment of weight, body shape and/or control over food

According to cognitive-behavioural theory, the central mechanism in maintaining DCA is a dysfunctional self-assessment scheme. DCA subjects have, like any other human being, a self-assessment scheme on which they base their sense of competence and effectiveness; however, if in other individuals this scheme mainly concerns some domains of life (such as work, sport, school, etc.), in DCA patients it is exclusively linked to weight, body shapes and nutrition control.

The extreme evaluation of body, weight and/or nutrition is, therefore, the mechanism primarily involved in the maintenance of NL; most other clinical features, such as compensation behaviour, dietary restriction, recurrent thoughts about weight, body shapes and nutrition or the avoidance of weighing and exposing one's own body18 , derive directly from it. Only the binge is a behavior that is not directly related to nuclear psychopathology and that manifests itself as a consequence of the attempt to tighten the diet or, in some cases, as a strategy to modulate emotions considered intolerable.

THE EFFECTS OF MALNUTRITION

Many of the characteristic symptoms of DCA are a consequence of unhealthy eating habits. By analysing their behaviour and personality, we can grasp three phases: one of regular nutrition (3 months), one of extreme dietary restriction (6 months) and, finally, one of re-feeding (3 months). In the restrictive phase there is an increase in hunger. With loss of control of the subject, increased obsession with food, decreased concentration and reduced sexual desire. A decisive change in eating habits. Therefore, having a restrictive and long-lasting diet becomes one of the negative and feedback feedback for subjects that flow into the DNA. Unhealthy eating habits increase, in fact, the concentration on food, body and eating; they aggravate the perception of one's own body image and internal signals; they trigger bulimic crises, due to the strong concern about control abilities, which in turn increase anxiety and fear of losing control; they reduce socialization; they increase emotional instability; they provoke a series of both physical changes (e.g., the loss of control of a person's own body image and internal signals). gastro-intestinal disorders, sleep disorders, decreased basal metabolism), both neuroendocrine and, by acting on the hedonic component of the diet (cognitive, emotional and linked to reward circuits), can lead to an increase in compulsive behaviour with respect to food and an increase in "addiction" eating behaviour.

Secondary gains related to the disease

Fear associated with sexuality, family conflicts, fear of getting fat, feelings of guilt and mood swings related to the effectiveness or otherwise of food control are negative reinforcements for people with NL. They, in fact, push the subject to focus on weight, body shapes and nutrition, allowing him to avoid the management of situations considered problematic. In the same way, the sense of triumph, mastery, self-control and superiority experienced after the use of compensatory or bulimic behaviors are positive reinforcements of a "cognitive" nature, which lead to live the conduct of elimination and binge eating, at least at the beginning, as protective and egosyntonic behavior. Social factors, such as compliments or attention from friends and parents, can also represent positive reinforcements.

These reinforcements, both positive and negative, last throughout the course of the disease and are an important maintenance factor, which in combination with other factors, determines the chronicity of the disorder (Balbo, 2017).

Events and emotions

People with NL often report frequent and intense emotions that they cannot tolerate; usually intolerance is towards negative emotional states, such as anger, fear, sadness, disgust, guilt and shame, but in some cases it is also observed towards positive emotional states, such as excitement. Rather than accepting and managing mood changes, these individuals can adopt dysfunctional and sometimes self-damaging behaviors in order to reduce emotional activation. Intolerance to emotions can, therefore, become a process of maintaining the eating disorder.

CHAPTER 2

EARLY TRAUMA AND NERVOUS BULIMIA: WHAT RELATIONSHIP?

The concept of psychic trauma occupies a central position in clinical theory and in the study of the pathogenesis of psychic disorders.

The first authors to deal with the concept of trauma were Sigmund Freud and Pierre Janet, who highlighted a direct connection between traumatic events experienced in childhood and mental disorders experienced in adulthood.

In particular, it was Janet's theories that increased scientific attention to trauma. During the last century, in fact, the role of trauma as the origin of disorders in children and adults has often been obscured or minimized, while in the last twenty years the importance that is being attributed to its effects on the physical and mental health of the individual is increasing.

Trauma, although originating outside the subject, draws its pathogenic power from its peculiar ability to alter the bio-psycho-social balance of the individual and to unhinge the mechanisms with which it interprets reality and gives it meaning. Trauma, especially if prolonged and experienced at an early age, tends to be structured as a "mental organization" and to be defined by characteristic affective states (anger, guilt, shame, impotence), pathogenic beliefs, relational styles, defenses, affective regulation modes and specific deficits of mental functioning. It, having a devastating impact on the developmental trajectories of the individual, can determine on the one hand alterations at the level of the body and its mental representation and, on the other, a weakening of the superior mental capacities, which, not integrating with the inferior functions, both for the input of information and for the behavioural output, can cause alterations at the level of the self-consciousness, of the memory, of the capacities of metacognition and of the regulation of emotions and impulses. These alterations, interfering with the adult ability to manage, process and deal with childhood traumatic experiences, can push the most vulnerable subjects to adopt dysfunctional behaviors of modulation of emotions, mainly of dissociative area, such as binge, self-harm (eg, cut off the skin) and/or the intermittent intake of psychoactive substances (e.g. alcohol or tranquilizers), which, having a role in the interruption of intrusive memories and in the modulation of anxiety and emptiness, can lead to the establishment of NL, creating a dangerous vicious circle.

MEDIATION FACTORS BETWEEN TRAUMA AND BULIMIA

Although traumatic events increase the risk of mental problems, many do not face any psychiatric problems. The correlation between trauma and subsequent development of the NL is, in fact, non-specific: "the existence of a specific and direct connection between sexual violence (or other traumatic experiences) and subsequent development of an eating disorder has not yet been demonstrated". Therefore, trauma is only a risk factor which, if related to other elements, can make the individual more vulnerable to the risk of developing psychiatric disorders, including eating disorders.

DISSOCIATIVE SYMPTOMS

Trauma, being an emotionally unsustainable event for those who suffer it, leads to the activation of archaic defense mechanisms, the famous four English F's, which cause detachment from the experience of oneself and the outside world and consequent dissociative symptoms, such as depersonalization and derealization. This detachment implies an abrupt suspension in the exercise of the normal capacities of reflection and mentalization and, therefore, an obstacle to the integration of the traumatic event in the continuity of psychic life.

Pierre Janet was the first, at the end of 1900, to study the relationship between traumatic experiences, dissociative symptoms and eating disorders. An essential concept of his theory is dissociation: a certain idea ("fixed idea"), or an entire complex of ideas and feelings that accompany it, escapes control and sometimes even the awareness of personal consciousness; this escaped or dissociated idea begins to live its own independent life and pushes patients first to refuse food, then to binge and, finally, to put it back without any control. Traumatic memories, therefore, are not removed from the consciousness but, from the beginning, are not integrated into the personal synthesis through the function of reality, leading, as a result, to the formation of real dissociated ego states, which can suddenly re-emerge alternating between them. According to the theory of the structural dissociation of the personality of van der Hart, Nijenhuis and Steele, within a traumatized subject there are two or more parts of the non-cohesive personality: an emotional part (EP), which is the one that lives at the time of the trauma, reliving it in an emotional and sensory-motor form, and that acts according to the biological system of defense; an apparently normal part (ENP), which is the one that keeps the memory inside.

The autobiographical of the individual, from whom, however, were excluded all the memories relating to the traumatic event and that allows you to live everyday life without feeling overwhelmed by the sense of emptiness and helplessness that would generate the memory of a painful event. These two parts alternate and, when the part detached from the trauma, operating through the systems of action of daily life, prevails, the subject appears rather serene and able to lead a normal life; However, if the emotional part prevails, then the person, vulnerable to the food disorder, can begin to experience an alteration of their body experience, which often results in derealization (feeling of unreality of the surrounding world) and depersonalization (a strangeness of their person, including the experience of their body) and live a series of dissociative symptoms, which can lead to the adoption of dysfunctional eating habits, in order to interrupt intrusive memories, modulate anxiety and fill the emotional void.

Dissociation manifests itself not only with the deficit of the superior integrating function, but also with the uncontrolled and disordered emission of the inferior one, no longer regulated by it ... Patients with BN often claim to assume a different personality during bulimic crises, as if they were possessed by a demon, or to live a sort of amnesia about what happened during the binge.

Therefore, according to the "mood modulation theory", dissociation could coexist with bulimic symptoms and have the function of reducing the intensity of negative affective states through experiences of detachment and transition to lower levels of consciousness; or in accordance with the "escape theory" could facilitate the triggering of binge eating, in an attempt to "escape" from the feelings of guilt and negative self-assessments compared to their perfectionist standards, through the shift of attention / consciousness from a more speculative and abstract level, such as self-assessment, to more immediate

46

somatic elements or external environmental stimuli, such as food.

Dysfunctional eating behaviors, in other words, as well as compensatory strategies, are experienced as a form of refreshment, nourishment, numbness, distraction, need for help, rebellion, liberation of anger, containment of sensory fragmentation and dissociation from intrusive thoughts, which in the long run can lead to the development of real psychopathological outcomes.

RISK OF RE-TRAUMATIZATION

Those who have been victims of unfavourable childhood experiences, such as physical and sexual violence, may be more vulnerable to subsequent stressful situations; in fact, one of the most surprising features of traumatised patients is the fact that they often find themselves involved in different circumstances in which the original traumatic situations or some of their elements are repeated.

Research suggests that many women, who have suffered violence during childhood, run a high risk of experiencing revitalization. This risk is lower in men, although it seems to be up to 5.5 times higher than in the general population. There is also a significant correlation between disorganised attachment and the reoccurrence of traumatic experiences. A possible explanation for this phenomenon may be the failure to learn to establish safe and appropriate boundaries in one's social interactions. The presence of seriously dysfunctional relationships with attachment figures has not allowed an adequate use of a "relational container" that serves as an opportunity for learning and integration of affective states. Moreover, most patients perceive themselves as bad and, because of this negative image of themselves, think they do not deserve anything positive, and end up resorting to the mechanism of dissociation as a defense strategy in subsequent stressful situations of life and/or as a strategy for structuring the personality.

Therefore, the presence of sexual or physical abuse in childhood makes it more than double the probability that a person is subject to at least one further abuse in the course of life. However, it is not only the repetition of sexual and/or physical violence that must be considered; other types of events may also occur between childhood trauma and the development of food-related symptoms, which may function as triggering factors in the development of childhood.

48

When the young adolescent is confronted with her sexuality and has more intimate contacts there are situations, even if positive and not at all violent, which can be experienced as traumatic and act in such a way as to arouse memories of traumatic experiences in childhood and the feelings and thoughts related to them have found that revitalization is associated with higher levels of eating disorders and impulsiveness.

NEGATIVE BODY IMAGE

Early mistreatment (sexual, physical and/or emotional), absence of protective factors and failure to develop age-appropriate skills cause a general "mortification" of the Self, which begins to be perceived as ineffective, powerless and unworthy, and this devaluation of the self-image also includes the image of one's own body; often, in fact, subjects with childhood traumatic experiences experience feelings of repulsion, disgust, hypercontrol and detachment from it. In such situations the problem is not so much the weight in defect or in excess, as the sense of one's own identity, because it is life itself, its meaning and value that have been transformed and altered. The body ends up becoming the most intimate and, at the same time, most alien representation of the individual, the inescapable scenario of all the psychic manifestations produced by the mind, the theatre where the game of identity is played.

The feelings of anxiety, embarrassment and shame in thinking that their physical appearance can reveal to others some personal inadequacies pushes subjects to adopt behaviors such as, for example, avoidance and denial of the body and compensatory strategies, which can increase body dissatisfaction and push them to focus more and more on controlling the weight and shapes of the body, giving rise to a real eating disorder.

Well, the negative body image can play a role as a mediator between the trauma and the NL: the maladaptive eating behaviors can, in fact, be interpreted as a "way to manage a negative image of himself and, more particularly, a negative body experience derived from sexual and / or physical violence.

CHAPTER 3

EYE MOVEMENT DESENSITIZATION AND REPROCESSING (EMDR) AND BULIMIA NERVOSA

EMDR, which stands for Eye Movement Desensitization and Reprocessing, is a new, standardized, eight-step therapeutic approach that aims to address the memory of the event and/or disturbing situation.

Currently, EMDR has been recognized as the most evidence-based psychotherapeutic approach to the treatment of Post-Traumatic Stress Disorder (PTSD) by the American Psychological Association and the International Society for Traumatic Stress Studies (ISTSS). However, EMDR, although in principle intended for the treatment of PTSD, is now also used for the treatment of other clinical disorders, including anxiety, somatization, dissociative, affective and eating disorders.

Psychological suffering, in fact, can assume many facets and, if for decades the world of psychology has focused exclusively on symptoms, in recent years is giving new importance to the difficult, stressful and/or traumatic life events that cause many psychiatric and psychological disorders.

It has been observed that many traditional therapeutic approaches do not place as a particular and primary focus on traumatic experiences, while EMDR Therapy is able to successfully address this limit. It, in fact, by synthesizing the elements of other effective psychotherapies, such as psychodynamic therapy, cognitive-behavioural therapy and therapy focused on the person and the body, with the characteristic elements of EMDR, such as short exposure to traumatic material or associated with trauma, bilateral stimulation of eye movements, awareness and free association, allows you to overcome the symptoms and go deep into the mechanisms of onset and maintenance of the disorder.

Its objective is to access traumatic memories and to carry out a rapid desensitization and a consequent cognitive restructuring of the experience of the individual.

EMDR, therefore, unlike other therapies, focuses on the memory at the base of the disorder and not on its consequences, so as to generate associations between previously fragmented information and develop new learning, which involves not only a reorganization of the personality, but also a change in the regulation of affections and other non-functional reactions.

The function of EMDR treatment is to free the patient from dysfunctional memories stored in memory and containing disturbing emotions and cognitions, proceeding from the inside out and dealing with the inner world before using tools and techniques to incorporate skill sets, which can characterize a healthy adult.

BIRTH AND DEVELOPMENT OF EMDR

The origin of EMDR occurred in 1987, following a random observation by Shapiro of the apparently desensitizing effects of spontaneous eye movements repeated on unpleasant thoughts: walking in a forest, the author noticed how the disturbing emotional component of some thoughts decreased rapidly and spontaneously as a result of the effect of sacchadian eye movements on some disturbing thoughts.

It was thanks to the discovery of this phenomenon that Shapiro started a work of about six months with 70 subjects on the use of guided eye movements;

what emerged from this study was, on the one hand, a significant reduction in psychic symptoms and, on the other hand, the definition of a standard procedure, called Eye Movement Desensitization (EMD), as it was thought, in accordance with its behavioral origins, that eye movements were specific in causing rapid desensitization.

With regard to EMD, in 1987 a controlled study was initiated on 22 subjects diagnosed with PTSD, which was subsequently published in 1989 in the Journal of Traumatic Stress; what emerged from this study was a significant change both in the levels of anxiety, which decreased, and in the number of positive convictions, which increased. This discovery led to a paradigm shift: it showed, in fact, the effectiveness of the EMD procedure not only for desensitization, but also for cognitive restructuring. What happened was, therefore, a change in orientation from an initial behavioral formulation, of simple desensitization of anxiety, to a more integrated paradigm of information processing.

EMD became EMDR, i.e. the word "Reprocessing" was added; this method, in fact, although it is better known and takes its name from eye movements, consists of many other components inherent in the clinical approach, protocols and procedures, which make it a more structured approach to psychotherapy. It has been observed that other forms of bilateral stimulation (e.g. hand drumming and auditory stimuli) can also be effective in information processing and that changes in the perception of anxiety and fear are the product of more complex cognitive restructuring. The EMDR, therefore, during its development, has evolved from a simple behavioral technique to an integrated psychotherapy approach with a theoretical model of reference: desensitization and cognitive restructuring can be considered as by-products of an adaptive reworking, which takes place at the neurophysiological level.

THE ADAPTIVE INFORMATION PROCESSING MODEL

The key theoretical principle underlying EMDR therapy is the Adaptive Information Processing model. According to this model, in each individual there is an innate system of information processing, which is configured to restore and maintain mental health in a manner similar to that of the rest of the body, brought physiologically to heal in case of injury. By storing the different experiences of daily life within a complex mnestic network, in which thoughts, images, sensations and emotions belonging to each single experience are integrated, it allows not only the adaptive resolution of the new incoming information, but also the development of new learning. "Memory is actually an active and dynamic reconstruction process influenced by both the initial engram (engram = the initial impact that an experience has on the brain) and other factors.

The pathology arises when this innate system of information processing is blocked: the mnestic components of a disturbing experience can, in fact, remain isolated from the rest of the neural network, without integrating with the other information. This lack of integration can lead to inadequate assimilation, which allows (whenever one is exposed to internal and/or external stimuli recalling the trauma) the emotionality and negative convictions linked to the traumatic memory of influencing the person in the present.

Therefore, when the innate processing system fails to integrate the information, it remains "blocked in the brain" in the same specific form it had at the time of input: the experience of a traumatic event and/or long unfulfilled interpersonal needs can, therefore, alter the biochemical responses (adrenaline, cortisol, etc.), which can block the innate brain system for information processing and leave isolated in a neurobiological stasis the information related to the trauma, thus compromising the mental health of the individual. What is created is a "knot", in which subsequent experiences, which seem similar to the first, are linked to the memory of the initial experience, remaining isolated from the remaining mnestic system of the individual and significantly hindering its functional behavior in the present.

It is clear, therefore, that in the AIP model clinical problems are considered linked to the memory of the individual's experience and that emotions, body sensations and dysfunctional thoughts associated with them are also a consequence of the memory, rather than a cause.

THE EMDR PROTOCOL

The EMDR protocol provides access to dysfunctionally stored information and the activation of the innate information processing system through bilateral stimulation, so as to store memories in a more adaptive resolution and create dynamic links within the mnestic network. EMDR procedures produce changes in the memory itself and in the way it has been stored: if before treatment a traumatic target memory manifested itself in a disturbing way and outside conscious control, after treatment this memory presents itself with less disturbing images, cognitions, sensations and emotions, demonstrating a shift of information from the non-declaratory memory system, or implicit31 , to the declaratory one, or explicit.

According to Siegel, unresolved traumatic memory is an explicit damaged process, in which there is no integration of the traumatic event within autonoetic knowledge. It is fundamental, therefore, at a therapeutic level, to retrace step by step the traumatic experience, as this allows to rearrange images, cognitions, feelings and sensations, and to make them part of the autobiographical narrative.

EMDR is a psychotherapeutic approach consisting of eight phases, each of which is formulated to strengthen the re-elaboration of dysfunctional stored information and learning. These phases focus on: past experiences that have contributed to the patient's current clinical condition; present events, which include current situations triggering the disease; and, finally, future situations that the patient would like to address with the desired attitude. They therefore provide a systematic way to explore and process negative experiences and to bring out the positive experiences necessary to restore a condition of well-being. By offering the possibility to consciously reflect on the traumatic experience, through the abreaction and the help of the therapist in his role as facilitator, they allow to explore the past cognitions, emotions and sensations and to assemble, even at a neurobiological level, the dissociative memories within the autobiographical narratives.

Here are briefly the eight phases of the standard protocol.

Phase one: patient history and information collection
The first phase of treatment with EMDR includes an assessment of the safety factors, i.e., your personal stability, the stability of your living conditions, the presence of stressors, your physical health and your ability to handle intense emotions.

Afterwards, the foundations are laid for the reception and construction of an appropriate climate of alliance and trust. In this phase we try to obtain a complete clinical picture of the patient, in order to realize an adequate therapeutic plan. This picture must include: the patient's life history, the history of attachment, the presence of traumatic events and memories related to them, the evaluation of past and present resources, the history of the disorder / symptom, the functional analysis of it and its current functioning.

The phase of anamnesis and evaluation, although it is carried out in most traditional psychotherapeutic approaches, in EMDR is of further importance: it allows, in fact, the identification of specific targets, which, if clearly defined, allow an effective initiation, processing and conclusion of treatment.

Phase two: preparation

The second phase includes the creation of a therapeutic alliance, the explanation of the process and effects of EMDR, the definition of a reasonable level of expectations, the management of patient concerns and the initiation of relaxation and safety procedures.

The objective of this phase is both to establish an adequate degree of trust between patient and therapist, and to prepare patients for the elaboration of specific targets, providing them with information and relaxation techniques, so as to increase their trust in the ability to handle high levels of disturbing material that may emerge during and after a therapeutic session.

The therapist should provide them with specific instructions: on EMDR therapy; on the functioning of eye movements and other forms of bilateral alternating stimulation; on the functioning of the information processing system; on the impact of traumatic events; on the possibility that unprocessed disturbing memories come to consciousness and may occur in the form of nightmares, new memories or flashbacks; and on the importance of giving precise feedback during the processing phase.

In addition to this, the therapist must teach patients relaxation techniques to manage any discomfort that may arise between sessions. A noteworthy technique is the visualization of a safe place, where the patient is asked to imagine a situation or a place that offers him a feeling of security, in order to generate, through eye movements (or other bilateral stimulations), emotional and physical feelings of relaxation.

Central to this phase is to give the patient the idea of feeling "in control" and at ease in the therapeutic situation and, in this regard, before starting work on the processing of information, it seems essential to verify the patient's ability to perform bilateral alternating stimulation. It is necessary, in fact, to use the type of stimulation most suited to the specific needs of the patient and, if the subject has difficulties with eye movements, other forms of stimulation can be used, such as drumming on the hands or sounds presented alternately.

In this phase, therefore, patients must perceive the therapeutic session as a "safe place" where they always have control of what is happening and can stop whenever they wish. Only in this protected condition, safe from the risk of re-traumatization, the EMDR intervention can focus on the disturbing memory to reactivate and complete the interrupted processing.

Step three: Assessment

In this phase the objective is to work on traumatic memories in a detailed and complete way and, therefore, to explore the primary aspects of each memory; among these: the image, the cognitions, the emotions and the physical sensations. For each memory, event or situation, identified in the first phase of the protocol, these individual aspects are analyzed.

Specifically, the first step identifies the target memory, on which you want to work and asks the patient to focus on an image that best represents him ("Which image represents the event?").

In the second step the patient is asked to verbalize the negative cognition (CN) about himself that emerges together with the disturbing memory ("Which words accompany the image and express his negative conviction about himself now?"). The term "cognition", although it is generally used to define all conscious representations of experience, is used in EMDR to indicate a belief or an assessment of oneself now, such as, for example, "I am powerless", "I am not worth it" etc.. The NCs, in fact, are records of the disturbing emotionality linked to the traumatic event and, in general, recall the sense of responsibility for the role played (weakness, inadequacy, etc..), the feeling of insecurity (of being exposed to danger) and / or lack of choice, which continue to affect the person in the present.

Thereafter, the therapist helps the patient to identify a desired positive cognition (CP), in which one would like to believe and which expresses a sense of control over the situation (empowerment) or one's own sense of value as a person ("When he recalls the image, what would he like to believe in himself now?"). The patient assigns a score to the CP to express how much he perceives it to be true for himself when it is related to the target situation. This score refers to the "Validity of Cognition/VOC", with a score from 1 to 7, where 1 is "completely false" and 7 is "completely true". This operation provides both the therapist and the patient with a baseline measure through which to see progress. It is also very useful to increase the patient's awareness of his cognitive distortions33 and represents the final destination, or rather the pattern of self that the patient would like to have once the therapy is over.

The patient is then invited to identify the emerging emotions, when the image and the CN linked to the memory of the trauma are combined ("When you think about the event and its negative cognition, what emotions do you feel now?"). The patient is asked to assign a score to the level of disturbance he is experiencing when accessing the memory, using the SOUTH scale (Scale Of Subjective Disorder Units/Subjective Units of Disturbance), which has scores ranging from 0 to 10, where 0 means "no disturbance or neutral" and 10 means "the highest disturbance imaginable". The assignment of this score allows to establish a subjective baseline measurement of the emotional reactions and, therefore, to increase awareness and to recognize the changes in the different emotions experienced during the session.

Finally, we focus on the body sensations related to the target through the body scan: the patient is asked to listen to his body and report in which parts he feels the feeling that accompanies the current reaction to the traumatic memory, on which one is focusing ("Where does he feel it in his body?"). This sensation is considered as a characteristic aspect of the memory itself, since the unprocessed memories remain stored at the body level; in fact, there is a somatic resonance to the unresolved thoughts and some studies have shown that, when a person experiences a trauma, the information and memories of the event are stored in the motor memory, rather than in the narrative memory, thus involving a constant experimentation of the same physical sensations experienced at the time of the trauma.

Phase four: desensitization

The objective of this phase is to access the target memory and stimulate the mnestic network, so as to allow the memory to connect to more adaptive networks.

During this phase of the treatment, the therapist invites the patient to keep in mind the selected image together with the NC and the relative sensation experienced in the body. Once the patient has focused attention on these target elements, the therapist invites the patient to let "whatever should happen, happen freely", while bilateral alternating stimulation is administered.

A bilateral stimulation set will then begin and after the first set, which usually consists of twenty-four bidirectional movements, where a right-left-right shift represents a movement, the patient is told to "erase everything and take a deep breath" and asked: "What do you notice now?". This question gives the patient the opportunity to report what he feels in terms of images, insight, emotions and physical sensations and, regardless of what emerges, the therapist invites him to focus on what he has reported, thus initiating a new set of bilateral stimulations.

This cycle of alternating focused exposure and patient feedback is repeated many times and is what allows proper processing of information quickly and effectively.

A processing is considered successfully completed when the "associative channel" of the target memory is cleaned and reclaimed and, therefore, when the patient no longer experiences disturbances and when no new disturbing elements appear after some control sets.

Since EMDR uses a non-directive method of free association, some people do not dwell on the details of the problem, but quickly and spontaneously access a succession of related thoughts, images, emotions, associations and memories. All this allows an adequate assimilation of adaptive information, found in other mnemonic networks, within the network that previously contained the isolated disturbing event.

The initial traumatic memory will lose, therefore, its pathogenic value and this phase can be considered complete when both the patient and the therapist will perceive an improvement.

Step five: Cognitive installation

The objective of this phase is to verify the validity of the positive cognition, previously elaborated in the assessment phase, and to increase its strength, in order to replace the original negative belief and increase the sense of self-esteem and self-efficacy in the patient).

The session begins with the therapist who asks the patient to remember the initial CP, asking if, in the meantime, another more suitable one has emerged.

67

During the desensitization phase, in fact, since the patient has the clearest and most
positive at its disposal, it may happen that new CP emerge that are more suitable from the therapeutic point of view or that the CP, previously developed in the assessment phase, is perceived as more truthful.

Subsequently, the patient is asked to focus simultaneously on the target, from which he started, and on the CP, thus proceeding with a series of bilateral stimulation sets

Step six: Body scan

The focus is on the body sensations experienced by the patient, when he thinks back to the target memory on which he worked. The therapist asks the patient to rethink the target together with the CP and to focus the attention on his body, from head to toe, in order to notice any signal, tension, rigidity or sensation arising from it. The information stored in a dysfunctional way can, in fact, remain at the physical level and this is indicative that the memory has not been processed in a way. It is therefore essential to carry out a body scan before the end of the EMDR session: if, in fact, during the scan, the patient feels tensions in certain parts of the body, he works on those sensations through bilateral stimulation. A memory can be considered integrated when both negative emotions and disturbing physical sensations disappear.

Phase seven: conclusion or closure

The seventh phase is the last phase before the end of the session and with it the therapist assesses both whether the material has been completely processed and whether the patient is in an optimal condition of balance.

It is essential to bring the patient back to a state of emotional balance by the end of each session and, if the processing of the traumatic memory has not been completed, the therapist can use the technique of the safe place, the techniques of self-control or guided imagination, in order to stabilize the patient and maintain a state of calm between one session and another.

In this phase it is important that the therapist deals with the patient's experience, provides him with further information, including realistic expectations about the negative (and positive) reactions that may arise after the treatment and, above all, explains what may happen in the following days: the processing of traumatic memories may, in fact, continue or other memories may emerge.

The instructions include an indication to keep a diary, which collects any emerging disturbance, such as flashbacks, thoughts, situations, memories, emotions or negative dreams, evaluating their disturbing level. All this will allow the patient, on the one hand, to provide a detailed report to the therapist in the next session and, on the other hand, to recognize their reactions, thus increasing their sense of mastery and knowledge of their emotions in various disturbing situations. The use of the personal diary allows, therefore, to create a sort of cognitive distance from emotional distress through writing.

Step eight: Verification or reassessment

Verification takes up the first part of each session after the traumatic memory has been processed. In this phase, the therapist: carries out a re-evaluation to record the effects of the previous session; ensures that all the goals achieved are stable and consolidated and that the CP is still perceived as true; listens to the story of what the patient has heard in the period between sessions; checks the diary kept by the patient to identify further targets; welcomes any difficulties experienced by the patient.

The re-evaluation is a very important phase, in which the therapist re-evaluates the elaboration of the

70

previously treated material and/or the possibility of turning to new disturbing material.

Fields of application of EMDR

EMDR is an elective therapeutic approach with people who are victims of specific critical events, caused by natural or man-made disasters, such as sexual abuse, domestic violence, combat, accidents, natural disasters and/or crimes.

EMDR, by favouring the activation of two brain areas, such as the front crawler and the left frontal lobe, allows not only the discrimination between real threats and trauma memory, but also the attribution of a meaning to emotions linked to traumatic memory, thus allowing the integration of memory into the flow of consciousness.

In recent years, EMDR has evolved into other clinical areas; research has shown the effectiveness and efficiency of EMDR not only in the treatment of PTSD, but also in the treatment of complex PTSD, anxiety disorders, body dysmorphism disorder, dissociative disorders, personality disorders, sexual disorders, substance use disorders, attachment disorders, somatization disorders and food disorders.

The EMDR procedures and protocols, in fact, being primarily an effective intervention on traumatic and/or stressful events, can be adapted to the peculiarities with which these events occur within the different psychopathological manifestations and personality characteristics. These experiences, in fact, rather than being connected in a privileged way to PTSD, seem to be considered transversal elements of psychopathology.

In conclusion, EMDR, starting from the assumption that the problem with which a patient arrives in therapy derives from traumatic experiences, can be used with different clinical and non-clinical populations (children, adolescents, adults), as well as in different areas: clinical, non-clinical and medical.

Food Behavioural Disorders from the perspective of EMDR

The theoretical perspective on which the EMDR therapy is based argues that the "causes" of the current symptomatology are to be found in past unprocessed experiences. Stressful life experiences and the resulting learning can, in fact, increase the development of numerous psychological disorders, including eating disorders.

Over the last decades, scientific research has shown significant empirical evidence on the link between eating disorders and traumatic event histories; the same DSM-5 has placed the emphasis on traumatic life events and, in general, on the interpersonal environment in the onset of the DCA.

Emotional and behavioural regulation, the ability to adapt and the consolidation of a stable and positive sense of self are, in fact, aspects strongly linked to the first relations with the significant figures. As the theory of attachment teaches, it is precisely within the first relationships with those who take care of us that we learn "who we are" and it is there that we build areas of strength, but also of vulnerability.

Consequently, a strong presence or, on the contrary, absence of such a link, if repeated over time, can represent a situation of threat, leading to a weakening not only of the superior mental capacities, but also of the inferior ones, generating a deficit in the regulation of emotions, impulses and behaviour.

In this perspective, food becomes something more than a simple object to eat; it is transformed into nourishment, refreshment, pleasure, bond, but also into damage and punishment. With respect to the latter, behaviour such as following a diet, bingeing and using laxatives, as well as the desire to be thin, although usually interpreted as a strategy to reduce anxiety, in the case of patients who have suffered unfavourable childhood experiences, in particular physical and/or sexual violence, can also be seen as a form of self-punishment or guilt. "Not eating can be a consequence of the idea that they must punish each other because they are guilty or because they are not good enough and do not deserve to give each other rewards". However, patients can resort to binge eating and compensatory conduct both to make their bodies sexually unattractive and, therefore, to protect themselves from possible future experiences of revitalization, and in a defensive way to avoid feelings, memories, feelings and knowledge related to the trauma.

Eating symptoms can, therefore, take on more functions and it is fundamental to try to understand what are the mechanisms that lead to the development of this disorder, what are the factors and stresses to which these patients try to react.

The EMDR therapy aims at this; its theoretical paradigm starts from the idea that symptomatic manifestations, including eating disorders, depend on past experiences.

traumatic events that trigger a pattern of behaviour, knowledge and emotions that cause a spiral of acute suffering. In this perspective, the symptoms of the eating disorder can be read as the result of a series of unprocessed and unresolved traumatic events and insecure attachments.

Post-traumatic affective regulation deficit
The term mentalisation was introduced into the Anglo-Saxon lexicon by Fonagy, who defines it as a form of imaginative mental activity, mostly of a preconscious type, which interprets human behaviour in terms of intentional mental states (e.g. needs, desires, feelings, beliefs, objectives, intentions and motivations).

Monitoring refers to the ability to distinguish, recognize and define one's internal states, i.e. cognitions, emotions and intentions, and the ability to establish relationships between mental variables, describing causes and motivations of one's behavior; differentiation refers to the ability to distinguish between different types of representation, i.e. dreams, fantasies, hypotheses, beliefs and between representations and reality, and to describe mental states and actions of others regardless of their point of life, without resorting to stereotypes or clichés; integration is the ability to construct coherent representations of oneself and the other, maintaining a sense of continuity as interpersonal contexts change; finally, the mastery refers to the ability to operate on one's own mental states to implement intervention strategies aimed at regulating and resolving states of psychological suffering, as well as interpersonal problems.

Studies conducted with brain imaging techniques have highlighted an interesting link between attachment and development of mentalization: this development occurs, in fact, in the first primary object relations and seems to involve different brain areas, including the pre-frontal orbital and medial area, mirror neurons starting from the premotor cortex, the structures of the temporal lobe (including the amygdala) and the temporo-parietal regions.

When, during childhood, psychological traumas occur, the normal development of mentalisation capacity may be compromised. Such impairment leads to a lack of self-reflection, that is, a difficulty in considering, reflecting and understanding one's own mental states and those of others, which can degenerate into a deficit in the possibility of regulating and organizing emotions, of understanding their contextual and transitory nature and of understanding the links between events and affections.

In recent years, some studies have dealt with the difficulties of mentalization and regulation of emotions in subjects affected by DCA. What emerged from these studies was that subjects who reported experiences of abuse in childhood, particularly emotional abuse, showed a higher correlation with the difficulties of mentalization and regulation of emotions.

With regard to the latter, empirical research in the field of DCA is numerous; most of these focused on the theoretical construct of alexithymia, which is related to the metacognitive function of monitoring and is understood as the inability to identify, understand and express their emotions and those of others. In patients with BN, alexithymia can be a stable trait of the personality and is linked to a sense of inadequacy and social insecurity, which can have a number of consequences on the level of emotional regulation: the reluctance to form intimate relationships and to communicate their feelings to others, and the difficulty in responding adequately to their emotional feelings and other aspects of the

77

experience of themselves. Moreover, according to some studies more inherent to trauma, alexithymia, besides being one of the most evident forms of metacognitive deficit, can also be considered one of the manifestations of dissociative processes that follow trauma. A controlled empirical study has, in fact, shown a correlation between alexithymia and dissociation, emotional dysregulation and somatization.

Also the disturbance of the body image present in patients with DCA can be read as a difficulty in adequately understanding mental states: Several studies have shown, on the one hand, how these patients attribute to others the idea that their bodies are unpleasant, in the absence of sufficient signs to indicate that others have such a perception, thus demonstrating a difficulty in decentralizing their thinking; on the other hand, how these patients have difficulty differentiating between their own subjective internal representations (e.g., sensation of swelling) and external reality, thus interpreting everything that is merely subjective as an objective fact. With regard to this last aspect, for example, many patients are convinced that they are fat (fantasy) in the presence of an objective comparison (actual weight) which contrasts with their belief.

Finally, studies conducted on emotional regulation have shown that DCA are characterized by problems in the regulation of affections, that is, the inability to use reasoning in mentalistic terms in order to regulate choices, to modulate negative emotions or to reach the solution of problems to face the psychological suffering that derives (Mastery). What immediately emerges from the clinical observation is, in fact, that in patients with DCA there is a low self-esteem and a tendency to evaluate negatively their own abilities and behaviors, leading to the fear of not being able to cope materially and/or emotionally with the dreaded situations. Such inability to carry out metacognitive reasoning related to the sense of self-efficacy would render the mind of these patients powerless and/or disorderly, leading to consequences on the level of emotional and behavioural regulation. An indication of this could be the binge, which is often preceded by strong negative affects, in which a pervasive sense of impotence and loss of control predominate; it could be interpreted as the behavioral strategy used to relieve emotional tension, given its direct action on the modification of the somatic state.

Bulimia as a dysfunctional coping strategy

When caregivers are abusing, absent, neglectful or helpless in the face of a traumatic event, children are not able to develop a sense of security and stability in their relationships with them.

The lack of sharing of affections, on which the child builds his experiences of self-efficacy and awareness, can lead to confusion about their mental states and can interfere with a normal development of the ability to regulate emotions, leading to both a constant activation and warning, and the adoption of dysfunctional behaviors.

A large number of studies on the etiopathogenetic factors of the NL have identified in pathological eating behaviours an attempt, even if painful and not very effective, of self-therapy.

The symptoms of Eating Disorders have an adaptive function of rest, numbness, distraction, sedation, energy source, need for help, rebellion, liberation from anger, sense of identity and self-esteem, maintenance of weakness/impotence, control and power, self-punishment and punishment of the body, containment for fragmentation and dissociation from intrusive thoughts. There would also be the functions of cleansing and purification, of escape from intimacy, as well as a strategy of coping to suppress the memories of the same traumatic experiences. Below I will examine how the main features of the NL are seen from the EMDR perspective.

Concern about weight, food and body shapes

The extreme concern for weight, food and body shapes is considered to be the specific psychopathology in subjects affected by NL; in fact, these subjects, having at the base a poor concept of self and a deep lack of confidence in the validity and reliability of their feelings, thoughts, perceptions and behaviors, believe that weight and fitness are of extreme importance to judge their value and that they should be kept under control.

From a cognitive point of view, the issue of control is closely related to the ability of internal states to regulate themselves and to the ability to influence external events. Therefore, it becomes extremely important not only in relation to food and, therefore, to the need to control its intake, but also in reference to all aspects that characterize the subject's daily life.

It is well known that the feeling of having control is associated with a state of psychological well-being, while the inability to exercise cognitive and emotional control can be considered a factor behind the onset of some emotional disorders.

In this sense, thinking about weight, food and body shapes is a coping strategy, an extreme and dysfunctional way in which the subject tries to reduce the negative idea of himself and his sense of vulnerability. Some girls report how the experience of "absence of feelings" is linked to a greater attention to weight, food and body shapes, or thinking about these external parameters allows them to distract themselves from the great inner void. However, it is also true that in people with bulimic behaviors there are high levels of impulsiveness, which decreases their sense of control.

The phenomenon of binge eating

The only behavior that seems not directly related to the concern for weight, food and body shapes is the one related to the binge.

An episode of binge eating is defined as the ingestion in a given period of time of a quantity of food significantly greater than that which most individuals would assume at the same time and in similar circumstances and is accompanied by a feeling of losing control, that is the feeling of not being able to refrain from eating or to stop eating once started.

This type of binge is called "objective", because the amount of food consumed during the episode is objectively high; this behavior should be differentiated from other very frequent forms of over-eating: the "subjective" binge, for example, is similar to the objective one except that the amount of food consumed is not objectively high. Moreover, not all individuals experience a loss of control; in some cases, binges can be planned. In line with this, what characterizes the binge is not the uncontrolled desire for a specific food, but rather the anomaly in the amount of food consumed. However, generally, during binges, "bad or fattening" foods are ingested, that is those avoided in the restriction phases, because they are considered caloric.

The individuals with BN typically feel ashamed of their problems with the alimentation and try to hide their symptoms; the binge eating happen in solitude and often continue, until the individual feels unpleasantly or painfully full. The most common antecedent of the binge eating is a negative emotion (anger, irritability, depression, loneliness, anxiety, guilt, sadness and worry). Other triggering factors may be: weight gain, which increases concern for weight and body shapes and thus increases negative emotions; the feeling of swelling and fatness, which is a typical state of mind in these patients; hunger, which can make it difficult to control nutrition and, therefore, facilitate loss of control; boredom; dietary restriction; stressful interpersonal conditions.

Before and during the bulimic attack some people report being agitated and experiencing a total lack of control over their behavior; others, however, report having an altered state of consciousness in the moments before and during a binge. In relation to this, some patients claim to assume a different personality and sometimes do not remember what happened, this is particularly frequent in patients with bulimic behavior victims of abuse experiences, where there are high levels of dissociation of consciousness (amnesia, depersonalization, derealization). These patients would resort to dissociation and, therefore, to binge eating, as a mechanism to manage the pain associated with trauma and to deal with the various stressful events of life. Such behaviour, in fact, produces at first pleasant sensations which, however, do not last long, giving way to feelings of disgust, guilt and self-devaluating depression.

There are two models that have tried to explain why binge eating occurs: that of food restriction and that of emotions. According to the model of food restriction, the binge eating would be the direct consequence of the strict diet: in most cases they occur, in fact, during periods of food restriction and may be induced by changes in hunger and satiety, from secondary emotions to food restriction or by the thought "all or nothing", typical of people with bulimia. However, this model has its limits: the first is that not all people who dabble restrict their diet before bulimic crises; the second is that the antecedents of dabbling are not always linked to stimuli of hunger and satiety, but also to negative emotional states or perceived threats to self-esteem. With respect to this last aspect, the model of emotions suggests two possible processes that could explain the link between binge eating and negative emotional states or threats to self-esteem: 1) the "process of blocking emotions", according to which binges have the function of distancing the individual's attention from emotional states perceived as intolerable; 2) the "process of escape from self-awareness", according to which binges are the consequence of a sort of cognitive restriction that the individual uses to escape from the awareness of negative emotional states or situations perceived as threatening.

However, the management of emotions through binge eating creates a sort of vicious circle: if, on the one hand, they can help to deal with negative emotional states and threatening situations in the short term, on the other hand, they do not put an end to the factors that trigger such problems. Moreover, it is often the binges themselves that have negative consequences, which in turn can trigger new bulimic crises.

The phenomenon of purging

Another essential feature of the NL is the frequent use of inappropriate compensatory behaviours; they are extremely important to reduce the feeling of physical discomfort, to manage the fear of gaining weight and, finally, to control the levels of anxiety (Dalle Grave, 1998; A.P.A., 2013).

People with BN, feeling unable to control their emotions, interpersonal relationships and life events in general, adopt behaviours of a controlling type, such as compensatory behaviours, in order to make their lives more manageable (Zaccagnino, 2017).

Self-induced vomiting is the most common compensatory technique used by these patients; its immediate effects are to reduce discomfort and the fear of getting fat (Dalle Grave, 1998). At the beginning, this strategy is experienced in a positive way as the solution of the problem, however, in the long term, it increases feelings of disgust towards oneself and one's self-esteem. According to some individuals, in fact, self-induced vomiting is a "not honest" weight control behaviour, which, despite this, is also used to manage events and mood changes.

In addition to self-induced vomiting, other elimination behaviours are used by bulimic patients, including the use of laxatives and diuretics, excessive exercise and a strict diet. With regard to the former, research shows that they are less frequent than self-induced vomiting: about one third of bulimic people use laxatives and only 10% take diuretics. They are used to eliminate excess calories taken during a binge and/or to exercise a form of control. Laxatives and diuretics can therefore be seen as an extreme and dysfunctional way in which the subject tries to control unpredictable events and threats from the surrounding environment.

Even compared to excessive physical exercise, research shows that it is less frequent in people with BN than in people with AN; in fact, it is typical in people with bulimic behavior to perform physical exercise occasionally. Like other compensatory strategies, excessive physical exercise can be a way to control and manage weight and body shapes, as well as events and associated emotions.

Finally, with respect to the iron diet, research indicates that it is a very frequent technique in people who suffer from BN. It, in fact, allows you to exercise control over what, how much, when and how to eat, thus helping to have the perception of some form of control over their lives.

All compensatory strategies can help to maintain the disorder and can be read as a dysfunctional coping strategy.

The role of traumatic memories and the maintenance of DCA

Taking up Janet's dissociative model, according to which dissociation is an idea or an entire complex of ideas and feelings that escapes the control and awareness of personal consciousness, it is possible to affirm that in patients with BN there can be "fixed ideas", unresolved traumatic memories, which lead patients first to refuse food, then to binge and, finally, to remit.

Traumatic memories, in fact, are not removed from the consciousness but, from the beginning, do not integrate into the coherent organization of memories and self-experience, leading to a disintegration with respect to the continuous flow of self-awareness.

From a neurobiological point of view, it has been seen how, in conditions of excessive stress, the amygdala, fundamental in the memorization of fear (implicit memory), does not persist in a deficit of memorization, unlike the pre-frontal cortex and the hippocampus, involved in the integration and evaluation of explicit memory. This involves the formation of intrusive memories, fragmented, not accessible to awareness and characterized by magmatic emotions, painful and difficult to manage, which can make more likely the development of psychic suffering.

In patients suffering from BN it has been seen how traumatic memories can contribute to the onset and maintenance of the disorder. They, in fact, can have a significant impact on the processes of information processing, on the processes of emotional regulation (rumination, avoidance of thought, dissociation) and therefore on the organization of DCA symptoms. In particular, it has been seen how traumatic memories related to feelings of shame play a central role in maintaining food symptoms. Shame, in fact, being an emotion with a negative value and deriving from unfavourable childhood experiences, can influence the well-being of the person, operating as a memory of intrusive self-definition and influencing the person's self-esteem and interpersonal style.

The first experiences of shame, having been stored at an implicit level, can suddenly re-emerge, generating reactions of anger, criticism and blame, which can lead to the adoption of eating habits, such as binge eating and elimination behaviour, in order to modulate such negative reactions and interrupt intrusive memories.

From this point of view, therefore, the traumatic memories and, specifically, the memories linked to shame, would act both as triggers (triggering cause) and as predictors and perpetrators of the alimentary symptoms.

EMDR TREATMENT IN THE TREATMENT OF BULIMIA NERVOSA

To date, we are not yet able to say what is the context and the type of therapeutic approach most suitable for a specific patient in a given phase of the disease. The international guidelines themselves argue that there is no specific type of treatment that can be recommended, as there are not enough studies about their long-term effects.

The field of research is still "behind" and, although Cognitive Behavioural Therapy (CBT) and Interpersonal Psychotherapy (IPT) are the most widely used therapies for the treatment of NL, other therapeutic approaches are gaining ground.

The research, having identified stories of unfavourable childhood experiences in a rather large percentage of patients affected by DCA, has paid attention to those forms of treatment that place a particular and primary focus on traumatic experiences. In particular, there has been a growing interest in EMDR therapy, which, having shown evidence of efficacy in the processing

91

and adaptive resolution of traumatic memories, has been used not only for the treatment of acute and chronic post-traumatic states, but also in those psychopathological situations, such as DCA, in which the body component is strong and a history of involvement in the development of the person is involved.

The EMDR, focusing on the understanding of the functional meaning of the eating symptom, allows to identify the mechanisms of onset of the disorder and to promote their reworking, overcoming, therefore, a purely behavioral perspective, to go deep into the mechanisms of onset and maintenance of the disorder.

Evidence to date in the literature shows that EMDR is a promising approach, which can lead to a resolution of traumatic and unresolved memories triggering food symptoms (Balbo, 2017).

The contribution of EMDR in the treatment of Bulimia

Away from Hudson, Chase and Pope's (1998) view that the use of EMDR in the treatment of DCA involves more risk than benefit, several studies have taken hold in the EMDR/DCA context.

The effects of EMDR on disturbed body image and low self-esteem were examined in a single case. The Daily Body Satisfaction Log was used on a scale from 1 ("very satisfied with my body") to 10 ("totally dissatisfied with my body") to record the body satisfaction of the 26-year-old patient in normal weight on a daily basis. The patient was instructed to assess her body satisfaction three times a day after meals for forty-three days. The Self-Esteem Rating Scale and the Body Image Avoidance Questionnaire (BIAQ) were used to assess self-esteem and pre-test and post-test body image. During the first session the woman performed the SERS and BIAQ as a pre-test; then she started the Daily Body Satisfaction Log for forty-three days, during which she underwent two EMDR sessions; and finally, at the end of the research, she performed the post-tests. The results of the research indicated a significant change in self-esteem, negative body image and levels of body satisfaction, recognizing, therefore, in EMDR an effective tool to improve the mental image of the body and self-esteem. Omaha, always through case studies, has conducted research in which he applied the EMDR protocol in the treatment of a bulimic patient. The results of the research have shown how EMDR can be a promising tool in the treatment of NL: it, in fact, working on traumatic experiences, allows not only the strengthening of resources, but also the disappearance of food symptoms. The effect of EMDR therapy on the so-called "emotional hunger" in a 55-year-old subject suffering from DCA. This study showed that there was a positive change in food symptoms and that, therefore, EMDR could be a valid tool for the treatment of "emotional hunger", understood as the regulation of emotions resulting from a traumatic history.

The results of the research showed that patients treated with both approaches reported less suffering with regard to memories of their body image and less bodily dissatisfaction after treatment in the following 3 and 12 months, compared to those who had received only the SRT. This research gave empirical evidence of how EMDR can be effective in treating specific aspects of DCA, including negative body image.

In conclusion, it can be said that although several studies suggest the efficacy of EMDR in the treatment of DCA, there are still no experimental studies (Balbo, Zaccagnino, Cussino et al., 2017). Most of the studies conducted have methodological limitations, such as the lack of a control sample and/or strict standardization procedures, which do not allow to generalize the results to the entire population (Ibidem).

Empirical evidence is being structured and, if EMDR is considered an evidence-based approach for the treatment of PTSD, further research is needed for DCAs. At a theoretical level, it can be argued that EMDR can improve food symptoms, emotional regulation, general well-being and mental health of the individual, thanks to its ability to actively intervene on traumatic memories, to lead to a resolution of unprocessed material, to access adaptive information related to disturbing memories and to decrease negative cognitions related to the sense of self-esteem and vulnerability. However, at the level of research, further empirical studies are necessary in this regard; the scientific literature, in fact, does not report specific studies on the treatment of NL with EMDR, while for the AN has already been conducted a controlled experimental study.

If for a long time it was considered that the work on the traumatic past was an essential element, a conditio sine qua non, of psychotherapeutic work with victims of trauma, in recent years it has been discovered that, for some patients, this work can turn into an experience of revitalization. EMDR, in fact, is not always a suitable approach; before starting work on trauma, it is essential that the therapist verifies, through an accurate medical history, the suitability of the patient for treatment.

First of all, in order to work with EMDR, it is important to verify the stabilization of the patient on a relational and personal level. With regard to the first aspect, it is necessary to assess whether the patient has adequate social support; the exploration of trauma requires, in fact, not only a certain strength on the part of the patient, but also the presence of social support outside the therapeutic environment. If the patient lives in isolation or does not have trustworthy relationships with other people, the EMDR therapy may not be indicated; in fact, it may involve a series of contraindications, which would cause more costs than benefits. With regard to the second aspect, it is necessary to assess whether the patient is physically and emotionally stable. Before starting work with EMDR, it is important to check the physical health of the patient and ensure that he has reached a certain level of physiological control, characterized by weight stabilization and a gradual reduction of symptoms. Also with respect to emotional health, it is important

96

to assess the stability of the patient, i.e. his ability to manage stress and control impulsive behavior, his ability to relax, the need for any hospitalization or drug therapy, the presence of dissociative symptoms and / or disorder in comorbidity. If, in fact, the patient is not emotionally stable, i.e. does not have management skills or attitudes to solve problems, EMDR therapy cannot be undertaken: the patient may present a (temporary) impediment to a direct confrontation with trauma, which would inevitably become a source of stress.

In addition to taking into account the patient's inter and intra-personal stabilisation, it is also important to assess the patient's motivation for change. Patients with DCA are often ambivalent to their willingness to undertake a course of care and change. "Several authors have described how patients with DCA have marked levels of resistance to change that often result in a lack of commitment to therapy. The psychological complexity of these patients, the interpersonal patterns dysfunctional, metacognitive and emotional modulation defects can prevent these subjects from adequately understanding and accepting the criticality of their condition, making them resistant (Ibid.). Some factors involved in the ambivalence towards therapy and change are: the desire to change only some of the pathological behaviors, such as egodistonic ones (e.g. binge eating) together with the strong desire to maintain others, such as egosintonic ones (e.g., the "binges"). The following are some of the most important factors: the lack of food restriction and the desire for thinness; personality characteristics, such as low self-esteem; affective-relational factors, such as the role of pathology in the modulation of relationships and emotions; socio-cultural factors, such as the emphasis that today's society places on thinness and social prejudice against overweight and obesity; finally, the phase of illness in which the person finds himself (initial phase or honeymoon, intermediate phase, advanced phase), which can influence attention to adaptive advantages or the loss of hope in the future. Therefore, before starting work with EMDR, it is necessary to assess the possible presence of secondary benefits, which are hidden behind the disorder presented. Patients affected by BN may, in fact, have organized their lives around the disease, it is therefore essential to work at first on building a therapeutic alliance, as will be explained below, and start work on the motivation for change: the latter, in fact, increasing the internal motivation more than the external and aspects that promote change more than maintenance, can promote more effective interventions and a better relationship between costs and benefits.

Objectives: present, past, future

One of the objectives of EMDR therapy is to start from the patient's life history and to bring out memories of traumas and/or critical events of the past, which have influenced the patient's self-esteem and prompted him to develop eating habits, in an attempt to compensate for the anxiety emerging from the trauma and to manage his emotional and affective needs. EMDR, by acting on the traumatic dimension, can reactivate traumatic memories related to the past and promote their association with the symptoms of the present. Possible work targets may be: attachment-related traumas, all situations in which the patient has identified an "attack" on the body and self-esteem, traumatic events (abuse, traumatic bereavement, accidents, etc.), as well as the first episodes in which food has been used in a dysfunctional way.

In addition to the past, through EMDR therapy it is possible to work on the psychopathological nuclei of the disease, representing the way it works in the present. In particular, the work on the present consists in focusing: on alimentary symptoms, that is on binge eating, on body image and on elimination behaviours, in order to facilitate the recovery of the most significant memories linked to the organization and maintenance of symptoms, not emerged during the analysis of life history; on negative beliefs of oneself, starting a process of cognitive destructuring; on the most destructuring emotions, such as shame, which, if focused, followed and desensitized, can dissolve an associative chain and lead to the re-elaboration of negative cognitions about oneself, which support the symptomatology (e.g., on the elimination behaviours, in order to facilitate the recovery of the most significant memories linked to the organization and maintenance of symptoms, not emerged during the analysis of life history). "I am ugly", "I am inadequate", "I am fat", "I am not lovable" typical of these disorders); on "slips" and on moments of impasse, which could occur during treatment. The main aim of the work on the present is, in summary, to allow the patient to process the symptoms and current difficulties, inserting and consolidating the contents learned during the psychoeducational phase, in order to strengthen progress and increase enterceptive awareness.

Finally, together with the work on the past and present, one of the objectives of EMDR is to conduct work on the future which, by strengthening the patient's resources, is very effective in removing symptoms and preventing relapses. This protocol, focusing on the image of the dreaded situation and the desired one, allows to identify the available resources, learned during the psychoeducational phase, and the positive contents, emerged during the elaboration of the targets of the past and present. This work is very important in the therapy with patients affected by DCA, whose treatment path is often characterized by relapses that, by reinforcing the negative beliefs of the patient with respect to the chances of recovery, interfere with the success of the treatment; therefore, the ability to make a protocol that aims to strengthen the patient's resources is useful in order to form new neural configurations, containing positive knowledge and more adaptive coping strategies.

The therapeutic relationship

Although some clinicians define EMDR as a method, as a monopersonal psychology, where the only person is the patient who performs a procedure, according to others the relational dynamics assume a central value in each of the eight phases of the protocol. EMDR is, in fact, a bipersonal psychology, where both the therapist and the patient are committed to building a therapeutic alliance, which acts as an emotional container for the processing of unresolved traumatic memories.

"Through each of the eight phases, the therapist is in relationship with the patient. The clinician has empathy for the patient. The clinician feels what the patient feels [...]. The clinician acts as a container and the patient has the opportunity to re-experience the trauma in the company of someone who takes care of it" (Dworkin, 2010).

When dealing with patients with DCA, the ability to build and maintain a good relationship is often compromised. The psychological complexity that characterizes these subjects appears, in fact, to be associated with important defects of metacognition and emotional modulation, with an inconsistent and fragmentary theory of mind, with frequent testing of the therapist, aimed at testing his availability, activating a mode of attachment sometimes "voracious", fragmentary, confused with other interpersonal motivational systems.

In accordance with the theory of attachment, entering into a relationship with the therapist implies the activation of the attachment system and the attempt to control or attack the therapist or to devalue or seduce him/her, far from being led back to the activation of other motivational systems, such as the competitive, exploratory or sexual system, can be read as an indicator of the establishment of a bond of attachment between the patient and the therapist and of the patient's resistance to change their interpersonal patterns.

"Before proceeding with EMDR, therefore, it is necessary to build the therapeutic alliance, to allow the patient to let himself be taken by the hand in the journey into the darkness of the disorder.

Although the therapeutic relationship is a crucial aspect of the EMDR procedure, it has a different value in relation to the phase of work in which the clinician and the patient find themselves: in the preparatory phases (Phase 1 and Phase 2) the importance of the relationship as an agent of change is low and the power of the therapist is high; during the active phases of the treatment (from Phases 3 and 4 onwards), the importance of the relationship increases and the power of the therapist decreases, passing from the role of expert to that of co-participant, in order to facilitate the re-elaboration of the disturbing state-dependent memories; finally, in the final phase of evaluation (Phase 8) the power of the therapist increases and the centrality of the relationship decreases.

Despite this different attention given to the relationship, it is, however, through it that the post-traumatic elaboration takes place, the management of the targets relative to the present and the installation of a future perspective.

The therapeutic relationship is, therefore, a crucial element for the success of the therapy; it, by increasing the mentalisation, favouring the expression and sharing of the emotional states, improving the efficiency of the metacognitive capacities of control of the emotions and of the behaviour, correcting the pathogenic beliefs hindering the relational life and increasing the personal synthesis of the subject, represents an opportunity of concrete emotional experiences, capable of correcting the deep regulatory schemes of the emotions, of the personal meanings and of the behaviour of the patient.

Since patients affected by NL tend to perceive the other in the relationship in an oscillating way, passing from an idealization of the therapist, perceived as indispensable and "decisive" for their own well-being in situations of "good relationship", to its devaluation, evaluating it as a deceiver and intrusive in situations of failure.

empathic, the purpose of the therapy is to encourage, from the first session, an accurate tuning between the clinician and the patient, as this is functional to the orientation of the evaluation of the patient as a confident partner or suspicious participant and, as a result, may allow a deeper healing or, on the contrary, superficial.

The importance of the safe place

When a therapeutic relationship with a traumatized client is established with EMDR, it is necessary that you anchor it in a secure relationship from the first session. Active work on trauma (Phases 3-6) can, in fact, only be successful in a safe atmosphere, where the patient no longer feels alone, the pain is shared and the necessary activities for accelerated processing of the information can be set. "In the first phase of the therapy the patient [...] needs to perceive the therapist 'on his side' to start building the safe basis that will support him throughout the therapeutic path".

The first step for a therapeutic relationship is a good working alliance, which implies the definition of the working objectives, the explicit understanding of the co-cooperation with respect to the shared tasks and the different roles and responsibilities of each one. However, this type of relationship, although a necessary condition, is not sufficient to work with traumatised patients.

As mentioned above, from the beginning of the therapy, the patient activates a style of distorted attachment, learned during his childhood; it is important, therefore, that the therapist places himself as a "safe base" in order to offer a resistant emotional container and allow the patient to trace in his memory those painful memories and express those emotions of anger, hostility, pain, fear, that in the primary attachment relationships had a distorted or deficient voice.

The function of the clinician is to maintain the patient's brain in a state of adaptive processing of information, supporting his processing skills and restoring the balance between excitement and inhibition. The other is seen as a person intelligent and worthy of consideration, able to make their own decisions and to initiate a personal process of self-healing.

The therapist's task is to work with the patient in a collaborative and coordinated way, being out of the process as much as possible; it is therefore fundamental that the therapist shows empathy, strategically transmits warmth, sensitivity, compassion, sincerity, honesty, great flexibility, commitment, acceptance and is attentive to how the patient lives the therapeutic progress and the role of the therapist in this process.

The therapeutic process is successful when it is assisted by the clinician, i.e. it is the patient's brain that is proceeding towards healing, while the therapist provides the structure and container within which this can happen.

Affective attunement can recreate the sense of patient safety and belonging through the dyadic relationship between patient and therapist. When the clinician chooses to be affectively tuned, in resonance and in alignment46 with the patient, he is creating something greater than safety: the attachment necessary to optimize the EMDR treatment.

The ability of the patient with evolutionary trauma to rely continuously on a care relationship is, in fact, compromised by the memories of traumatic relationships that the patient relives during the interaction with the therapist (Liotti & Farina, 2011).

One of the tasks of the work with the EMDR is, therefore, to identify possible breakages, prevent or talk about them, manage the transference and countertransference, in order to ensure the establishment of a bond that creates optimal security between the two people, in which the therapeutic process must take place. If, in fact, the patient enters into resonance with a different mental model of the "other" including, may be more likely to connect with the clinician in a different way than his attachment figures. This allows a new management of fear, which is no longer based on the defensive exclusion of information that would lead to painful emotions. Defensive strategies are replaced by elaboration processes that are no longer prejudicial and by emotional and behavioural responses adapted to reality. If the patient does not feel safe or ready to elaborate a memory, co-regulation takes shape, communication continues in a collaborative way and, through the common work on stabilization strategies, the return to affective tuning is encouraged.

"Retrospective reflection on past experiences is an important element, but very often (or perhaps always) not sufficient, in the therapeutic path to change. The direct and immediate experience of emotional experiences and reciprocal reactions in a new interpersonal context, such as the therapeutic relationship - an experience in which new ways of interacting with others are tested - is sometimes the first step necessary for a path that, even before full awareness, allows the patient to move in the direction of a cure" (Liotti & Monticelli, 2014).

THE PREVENTION OF THERAPEUTIC DROP-OUT

In the treatment of DCA, the therapist is often faced with a non-cooperative attitude or a clear rejection of the therapeutic intervention. Treatment compliance is often difficult and the risk of therapeutic drop-out is frequent. With regard to this aspect, in the international literature, the extent of the phenomenon varies between 20 and 73%, with an average value of around 13%. Mahon (2000), in a study on the drop-out of patients with DCA, revealed a variable treatment abandonment rate.

The causes of the phenomenon are many and can be referred to both the patient and the therapist: an early drop-out is more correlated to the presence of factors involving the patient and his attitude towards therapy50, while a late drop-out seems to be more correlated to the lack of sharing of objectives, to therapeutic errors, to the therapist's excessive technicality and to the ineffectiveness of the therapy. As far as this second aspect is concerned, many patients declare that they have abandoned the treatment due to misunderstandings with the therapist and disagreement towards the therapy both with respect to technical aspects, such as the compilation of the food diary (32%), and with respect to relational aspects, such as the detachment and coldness of the therapist (26%).

With respect to the correlation between therapeutic alliance and drop-out, it emerged that it is the fragility of the relationship between patient and therapist that plays an important role. Research has shown that, in the treatment of DCA, it is the quality of the relationship between patient and therapist that represents the most predictive therapeutic factor of the treatment outcome. The most positive aspect is recognized in the therapist's ability to build a "good therapeutic alliance "51 and, therefore, in his capacity for empathy, mentality, availability and interest in treatment and assumption of supportive and collaborative attitudes, as well as in the type of therapeutic technique used. The construct of "therapeutic alliance" has assumed, for most of the psychotherapeutic orientations, a transversal importance and the same EMDR therapy, although it has its roots in the background of cognitive-behavioural therapy, gives a fundamental value to the relationship.

EMDR is, in fact, a highly interactive approach, which requires sensitivity and flexibility on the part of the therapist, as well as good clinical judgment. Such an approach should not be conducted in the absence of adequate patient history, treatment plan and good patient-therapist relationship.

With patients with BN, moments of impasse are inevitable steps in the therapeutic process. Responding to these phases of breakdown with attitudes rigidly adhering to the therapeutic protocol, imposing on the patient what is considered a good

111

EMDR practice, could entail the risk of no longer listening to the patient and of further worsening the therapeutic alliance.

It is fundamental, therefore, to remain focused on the patient and the relationship, as this allows to maintain or restore the spontaneity of the relationship and, therefore, to promote the therapeutic alliance, essential to prevent the drop-out.

CHAPTER 4

THE OTHER DCA: ANOREXIA AND BED

ANOREXIA

Often the premorbid personality of anorexics is characterized by introversion, low self-esteem, perfectionism; in many cases there is a higher than average school performance, attributable to an intense commitment to study rather than to a high IQ. Vague digestive disorders are often cited with the aim of limiting the intake of the food proposed; at other times patients discard the food given by hiding it or throwing it away. Subsequently, the search "at all costs" for thinness with the elimination of foods with higher calorie content and standardization of a minimum and insufficient diet becomes more evident. Behaviors are often ritualized to increase energy consumption, with unusual hyperactivity contrasting with slimming.

Most patients are hungry but deny it. Often the desire for food re-emerges in the form of bulimic crises: real binges that end with self-induced vomiting.

The disturbance of the body image, which can even take on delusional characteristics, is accompanied by the denial of disease and the consequent refusal to cure oneself.

Criticism and pressure from the environment (almost always the family environment), aimed at obtaining a correct diet from the sick, instead, strengthen the intentions of fasting. The expiry of the general conditions is accompanied in many cases by the appearance of depressive episodes.

In the advanced phase of the pathology the following may appear: sleep disorders (difficulty in falling asleep and early morning awakenings); restlessness; inability to concentrate.

The disorder needs immediate treatment to prevent the tendency to become chronic.

Hyperactivity, the search for thinness and phobia of weight, the absence of delusions of venephibia and bizarreness of the diet distinguish Mental Anorexia from secondary wasting to organic diseases, the lack of appetite in depression and schizophrenia.

114

As for the course we can say that often it is a single episode followed by remission but the disorder can assume recurrent characteristics.

Mortality is around 5-20% due to malnutrition and electrolyte imbalances.

The therapeutic intervention is difficult to carry out with the anorexic patient not motivated to a healing process.

The choice of therapy must be early and oriented not to neglect the factors of maintenance and chronicity that can lead to death (diet, weight loss, excessive concern for body shapes).

Immediate should be the interim evaluation aimed at correcting dehydration and electrolyte imbalance.

Hospitalisation is recommended and becomes essential if the following conditions are met:

weight loss > 25% of the ideal weight
serious organic complications
risk of suicide
to move away from the socio-family environment.

The effectiveness of drug therapy (antidepressants if there is depression, antihistamines to promote appetite), psychodynamics and family depends on proper nutritional education.

Anorexia Nervosa generally requires longer treatments than Bulimia.

Anorexia nervosa is the eating disorder commonly associated with emaciation and excessive exercise. The onset is often linked to a stressful event and generally occurs during adolescence or early adulthood. It manifests itself with marked obstinacy in maintaining body weight below the

threshold of normality and health, dismayed by an intense fear of regaining weight or fattening. People tend to avoid foods with a high nutritional content, preferring low-calorie and water-rich foods. Very often, food restrictions are accompanied by self-induced vomiting and the use of laxatives or diuretics, while other times they result in actual fasting. Sometimes even drugs can be used improperly, for example by manipulating the dosage. Self-esteem and self-assessment are based primarily on body weight, but a distorted view and perception of one's physicality leads individuals to feel 'too fat' all the time. The severity of the disease is understood by both functional disability and body mass index (BMI). The latter identifies four different ranges, giving a 'mild' grade if below 17 kg/m², 'moderate' and 'severe' if within the 16.99-15 kg/m² range, and 'extreme' if below 15 kg/m². Among the most reliable diagnostic markers are amenorrhoea, lethargy, hypothermia, bradycardia, hypotension and cold intolerance. Despite the heavy weight loss, most anorexics do not recognize the seriousness and danger represented by the latter. On the contrary, for many anorexics it is important to continue to lose weight and body checking is a repetitive dysfunctional control behavior with which they ensure to continue in accordance with their goal. They can weigh themselves assiduously and continuously, measuring the circumference of the waist and thighs multiple times a day and using the mirror persistently to control those parts perceived as 'abundant'. Compulsive symptoms are in fact a common feature of these subjects and often become more pronounced with the continuation of the disease. Mental rigidity, reduced social spontaneity, feeling of inadequacy and repressed emotional expressiveness are the most common characteristics. In addition, it is important to remember the high probability of psychiatric comorbidity; the pathologies generally associated with anorexia are major depression, obsessive-compulsive disorder, other anxiety disorders and dependence on alcohol and substances.

BINGE-EATING DISORDER OR UNCONTROLLED POWER SUPPLY DISORDER (BED OR DAI)

I felt my stomach would explode at any moment.
other than that, the heart was beating fast because of
work overload,
His tongue swollen, and I felt faint.
(Anonymous)

In the fourth edition of the DSM, uncontrolled eating disorder was included in the category of Not Otherwise Specified Eating Disorders (NAS or EDNOS in English terminology), which included all cases that did not meet the criteria of any other specific eating disorder. Subsequent studies have highlighted the high incidence rate of this disease and have highlighted the need for further study of this issue. In the fifth and last edition of the DSM, in fact, the uncontrolled eating disorder is identified as a eating disorder in its own right, with well-defined diagnostic criteria and differentiated from the disorders listed above. Although clinicians are aware of this, there are still some fallacies related to the identification and diagnosis of the disorder, which according to the study by Supina and collaborators, can be overcome through detailed knowledge of the patient's history and specific questions about eating behavior. The main feature of uncontrolled eating disorder is the presence of recurrent binges, which must occur, on average, at least once a week for three months. These episodes occur hastily and mechanically, sometimes without even chewing food, and strictly alone, away from prying eyes. This sense of 'hunger' is not given by a real nutritional need, but often comes from a feeling of frustration that evolves into a frantic and desperate search for food. The individual eats until he feels unpleasantly full, and only at that point comes a strong sense of helplessness and inadequacy. Unlike bulimia, however, the episodes of 'compulsive feeding' are not followed by compensatory practices. This is the reason why the person with an uncontrolled eating disorder tends to gain weight and, therefore, to be obese. The subjective evaluation of the day affects the frequency of binges: the more the individual perceives the situation in which he is involved as stressful, the more the binges will be numerous and caloric. The minimum number of weekly binges to meet the criteria of the DSM-V is one, and up to 3 episodes per week the disorder is defined as 'mild'. From 4 to 7 episodes the severity is 'moderate', while it becomes 'serious' in the true sense of the word when it reaches 8-13 episodes per week. In the so-called 'extreme' cases, the frequency is even higher than 14 episodes per week (DSM-5). A typical feature of patients with uncontrolled eating disorder is low self-esteem, in fact they are often involved in a vicious circle whereby failures of dietary regimens facilitate the relapse into binges and contribute to the further worsening of self-esteem. Significant psychiatric comorbidities are associated with anorexia and bulimia, with a higher probability of bipolar disorder, depressive disorder, anxiety disorder and, to a lesser extent, substance use disorder.

NEUROSCIENTIFIC EVIDENCE OF EATING DISORDERS

Eve's fault was that she wanted to know, experiment, investigate with her own strength the laws that govern the universe, the earth, her own body, to refuse the teaching from above, in a word Eve represents the curiosity of science against the passive acceptance of faith. '

Margherita Hack, Free science in free state

The scientific evidence at the neurobiological level seems to be consistent with the clinical and diagnostic models explained in the previous chapters. The salient aspects at the psychological level are confirmed in recent studies of neuroimaging and neurobiology. To date, the techniques mainly used to investigate eating disorders are those of anatomical neuroimaging (magnetic resonance imaging) and functional neuroimaging (single photon emission SPECT-tomography, positron emission PET-tomography, functional magnetic resonance imaging). Recent studies have made an enormous contribution not only to the diagnosis of diseases, but also to the development of therapies that, although intrinsically relational, are making use of the strength of scientific evidence in the design of treatment tools. This paragraph therefore aims to review some of the recent neuroscientific evidence found in eating disorders.

REDUCTION OF THE VOLUME OF GREY MATTER

Already the first studies carried out on patients with eating disorders showed the existence of significant and characteristic brain changes. For example, Dolan and co-workers (1998) had found an overall decrease in grey matter in anorexic patients, accompanied by larger ventricular zones and more pronounced grooves, compared to control subjects. More recent research has instead focused on more specific brain areas. Castro-Fornieles and co. (2009) found, in 12 anorexic patients, both a global reduction in brain substance and a more severe decrease in particular areas, such as temporal and parietal areas. Moreover, the grey matter (formed by neuronal nuclei) seems to be more affected than the white matter (myelinated axons of neurons) and can be partially recovered after weight recovery. Joy and co. (2011) confirmed, in their study, the presence of global cerebral hypoperfusion, including all gray matter. In addition, they found that the most affected bilateral regions were those of the medial cingulate cortex, precuneus and lower and upper parietal lobes. The neurons of the girdle gyrus, which are part of the prefrontal cortex, seem to have a wide role in cognitive processes of different entities. They contribute to the processes of reward, performance warning, control and selection of actions. They could also have an integrative role of all these capacities, summarized in the function of 'allocation', understood as the distribution of control. The precuneum is instead located in the parietal lobe and is also involved in various integration tasks. It contributes to the elaboration of visual-spatial information, to the recovery of episodic memories and to the development of the Self, to the personal perspective of events and to the sense of first-person 'action'. The lower and upper parietal lobules are responsible for sensomotor integration, estimating the state of the external world and that of the body. The areas described above collaborate in the construction and manipulation of mental images, in the mental representation of oneself, and in personal awareness. Their malfunction would explain the distortions of the self-image found in patients with eating disorders.

In bulimic patients with uncontrolled diet, few studies have been carried out to detect abnormalities of the brain substance. One of the first investigations, conducted by Hoffman and co. (1989) on people suffering from bulimia, noted a widespread cerebral atrophy, but did not detect a magnification of the ventricular zones. Woolley and collaborators (2007) found a strong correlation between frontal atrophy and binge eating behaviour. More precisely, the damaged areas are those related to the orbitofrontal-insular-striatal circuit, which already previous neurophysiological studies, in humans and non-human, had identified as a contributor in the regulation of eating behavior. In contrast to these data, a neuroimaging study conducted by Shafer and co. identifies an increase in the volume of the orbitfrontal cortex in people with bulimia and uncontrolled eating disorder. The high reactivity of this area can be interpreted, according to the authors of the research, as the explanation of the dysfunction of the processes of reward (hedonic mechanisms) and self-control.

FRONTAL LOBE

One of the first studies conducted by Nozoe and co. found greater prefrontal activation, when anorexic subjects were eating a cake, compared to the resting condition. Subsequently, several functional neuroimaging studies investigated the frontal lobe response of people with eating disorders. A study conducted by Uher and co. (2004) on subjects with anorexia and bulimia, found that visual stimuli associated with food are evaluated as significantly less pleasant, and indeed, more disgusting and frightening, than neutral stimuli. In addition, the left orbitfrontal cortex and the cingulate cortex, brain areas responsible for processing emotional information and related to the onset of obsessive-compulsive diseases, with which eating disorders often overlap, were found to be more active than control subjects. This anomaly, found in anorexics and bulimics, can be considered as a neuronal substrate common to the two diseases. The same study also identified a particular deactivation of the anterior and lateral prefrontal cortex in subjects with bulimia. Occurring in conjunction with food-stimulants, and knowing its main role in suppressing unwanted behavior, the authors associated its decreased activity with loss of inhibitory control and episodes of binge eating, found in these subjects.

Two studies seem complementary in deputing a fundamental role of the medial prefrontal cortex in the concept of body image in eating disorders. Patients with anorexia, when exposed to images of body monitoring actions (such as weighing or measuring circumferences), show reduced activation of the medial prefrontal cortex and right fusiform gyrus, in conjunction with higher levels of anxiety than control subjects. These areas are generally activated both in the elaboration of external information that has to do with one's own person, and in the recognition of emotions and intentions in the bodies of others. This result has been interpreted as evidence of the difficulty of anorexics in perceiving actions of their own body and with reference to themselves or others of the perceived stimuli. Even those who suffer from bulimia seem to run into problems in the personal attribution of images observed. In a study by Spangler and Allen, experimental, bulimic and control subjects were exposed to the vision of lean bodies and fat bodies. In people with bulimia, in the first case there was a normal activation of the medial prefrontal cortex. In contrast to this, there was a significantly higher activation in the second case, corresponding to the subjects' conviction of being overweight.

REWARD CIRCUIT

The 'circuit of reward' is so called because it acts in the sensations of gratification and satisfaction. Patients with anorexia practice physical exercise in a compulsive and systematic way, and find satisfaction in activities that directly or indirectly concern weight loss (DSM-5). The fact that the feeling of gratification comes exclusively from certain activities has suggested the hypothesis that, in anorexic patients, there are alterations in the circuit of reward. Kaye and co. found a lack of dopamine and a consequent dysfunction of the reward system, both in anorexic subjects under treatment and in the remission phase. Other neurobiological evidence shows a hypo-activation of the reward circuit in patients with bulimia. The study by Volkow and co. (2009), which investigates the role of dopamine in the abuse of drugs and other addictions, reveals that a deficit of this neurotransmitter is related to loss of control and compulsive use of drugs. The decrease in dopamine may also reduce the sensitivity to natural reinforcements. Based on the above study, and given the similarities between bulimia and substance addiction disorders, Broft and co. (2011) investigated the concentration of dopamine in bulimic patients. In comparison with control subjects, a lower dopamine release was found in bulimic patients; moreover, this release is significantly and negatively associated with the behavioral responses of binge eating and compensation. The 'hypo-responsiveness' of the reward circuit may suggest that in bulimics, compared to control subjects, a greater amount of food is needed to satisfactorily stimulate this circuit. This would result in a continuous search for rewards and loss of inhibitory control.

SEROTONERGIC CIRCUIT

Studies of the serotonergic system in anorexic patients have shown that the abnormality of this neurotransmitter contributes to the promotion of symptoms of the disease, increasing the sense of satiety and control of impulses. Bailer and collaborators (2007) found an increase of this substance in relation to the presence of anorexia, deputing this increase as a compensatory response to lack of food. However, the role of this transmitter in the pathology in question has not yet been precisely identified.

The dysregulation of serotonergic activity in bulimia can be related to the impairment of inhibitory control over food intake. In fact, a reduction in serotonin correlates with an increase in food intake and corresponds to an irritable mood in patients. To confirm this, bulimics respond to the administration of selective inhibitors of the reuptake of this neurotransmitter with a reduction in the frequency of binge episodes.

INSULAR LOBE

When food is introduced into the mouth, the tongue receptors detect the taste and send the related sensory information first to the thalamus, then to the insula (primary gustatory bark). From the latter depart several connections with the amygdala, the anterior cingulate cortex and the orbitofrontal cortex (secondary gustatory cortex); a greater activation of these indicates a sense of pleasure given by food. Given the primary function of the insula in processing gustatory messages, Kaye and collaborators (2010) have examined the activation of the same, in anorexic patients. The results showed a hypactivation of the island lobe with a consequent decrease in the other areas involved. From this could derive the feeling of poor appetibility of food and weak appetite, explaining how it is possible, for some, to prolong the emaciation until death. In addition, the insula is involved in enterceptive processes, contributing to the awareness of body states. Some clinicians have hypothesized that its alteration could result in ambivalent and confusing body sensations. Examples include obsession with food and cooking in the absence of appetite, distorted body image and poor motivation to change, or inappropriate methods of coping with hunger (Kaye et al, 2010).

CONTRIBUTIONS

New methodologies of neurobiological investigation can make a huge contribution to the treatment of eating disorders. A first contribution is given by the increase of the knowledge of the pathologies, thanks to the more precise and structured identification of the symptoms that characterize the eating disorders. A second element is defined by the improvement of the effectiveness of existing pharmacological treatments, which currently cannot boast of constant and significant effects. The main contribution, however, is made in supporting the design of therapeutic techniques. Thanks to the precise identification of the neuroatomic bases involved in the etiology of eating disorders, a more effective use of neuromodulation techniques (SMT) or similar techniques will be possible in the near future. A better understanding of brain circuits and hemispheric connections is instead to support the new and efficient techniques of Desensitization, such as EMDR therapy (see next chapter). In addition, it is necessary to mention the importance of the results of neuroimaging studies in the design of adequate therapeutic treatment and the monitoring of its medium- to long-term effects.

CHAPTER 5

WHAT IS MUSIC THERAPY?

HARMONY HEALS THE SPIRIT AND ALSO THE BODY.

Producing and listening to notes, sounds and melodies eliminates energy blocks and helps to regain serenity: here is a brief introduction to music therapy.

Music has always cared for. Its enchantment and therapeutic powers have grown with human consciousness.

Even the primordial sounds, produced by improvised instruments such as a trunk, a drum, wood beaten against each other, in the past had particular effects on the psyche, healing some diseases of primitive peoples, contributing to the social interaction between members of the same tribe, bringing our ancestors to higher states of perception.

Today, those same beneficial consequences of rhythm and melody have taken the name of "music therapy".

This application of notes to medicine, which requires precise techniques and a structured approach to the patient, has a recent history instead.

Music therapy was born as a specific discipline between the end of the nineteenth and the beginning of the twentieth century, with the sending of some musicians in American and European hospitals to give relief to the suffering by supporting the morale on the ground. Later - during the Second World War - in the United States the first interventions of therapy with music with groups of veterans were experimented. The accumulated experiences have led, in a very short period of time, to the development of numerous music therapeutic techniques and real methodologies.

Today we have different and numerous definitions of music therapy; according to the Canadian Association of Music Therapy, the latter is "the use of music to promote the physical, psychological and emotional integration of the individual, as well as the use of music in the treatment of diseases and disabilities. It can be applied to all age groups in a variety of care settings. Music has a non-verbal quality, but offers a wide range of verbal and vocal expression.

134

The World Music Therapy Federation defines it, however, as "the use of music and/or musical elements (sound, rhythm, melody, and harmony) by a qualified music therapist, with a client or group, in a process that facilitates and promotes communication, relationship, learning, motor skills, expression, organization and other relevant therapeutic objectives in order to meet the physical, emotional, mental, social and cognitive needs".

There are different methods to cure with music, more precisely different music therapy techniques, precisely "active and/or receptive" and "individual and/or group".

Both active and receptive music therapy arise in some way from the failure or inadequacy of verbal mediation. Both interventions therefore have their own specificity in clinical contexts where it is necessary to establish a contact, an approach. This is proposed through a gratifying sensory-perceptive solicitation, in the active approach, or through a metaphorical psychic nourishment in the perceptive one.

Turning instead to the indications relating to individual and group treatment, it is clear that the first indication on the subject arises also in this case from clinical considerations; these may suggest the choice of an individual or group context in relation to the potential and needs of the patient. In addition to this, in order to address ourselves in one direction or another, we will take into consideration the qualities of the relationship that the patient establishes with the sound/musical element and its introspective, introspective and processing skills. The more the relationship that the patient establishes with the sound/musical element appears to be specific, deep, peculiar, the more it is possible to hypothesize an individual assumption of responsibility; vice versa, the more this relationship appears generic, superficial if not defensive, a group treatment can be hypothesized where these aspects can benefit from the comparison with the others.

The music therapist tries to understand what the needs of the patient are, decides the approach and the individual program to follow and then chooses specific musical activities to achieve the goals.

Music therapy has a complete approach, embracing the individual in all his parts, which wants to recognize and develop internal resources, often not exploited.

Music becomes "clinical improvisation", that is, a flexible sound language that develops moment by moment on the basis of the careful and continuous observation of each patient who, in turn, lives an experience so intense from an emotional point of view as to be able to transfer it into daily life.

The basic principles of this line of thought are: clinical improvisation, use of various instruments, wind, string and percussion, sound dialogue and vision of man according to the conception of humanistic-existential psychology.

Music therapy is, therefore, a new specialist branch, whose scientific bases, on a clinical-therapeutic level, are sufficient to establish a clear working methodology and a set of techniques that can be developed.

Music therapy, in its clinical application, must be practiced exclusively by a music therapist (expert).

Music therapy cannot be improvised and, since it is a scientific discipline, it has such deep incidence possibilities that, if practiced by a layman, it can easily give rise to iatrogenic effects.

The term music therapy is, in fact, very ambiguous because it is applied to a specialized field that uses a whole series of phenomena not precisely related to music proper: in fact, there are also sound, noise, movement, etc., and essentially all this is summarized in one of the non-verbal therapies par excellence.

According to R. Benenzon, music therapy can be defined essentially in two ways: one considers the scientific aspect, the other the therapeutic one. From a scientific point of view, music therapy can be defined.

"A scientific discipline that deals with the study and research of the human sound-being complex (musical or nonmusical sound) with the aim of researching elements of diagnosis and therapeutic methods".

From the therapeutic point of view, instead, music therapy is

"a discipline that uses sound, music, and movement to cause regressive effects and open channels of communication, with the aim of activating, through them, the process of socialization and social inclusion.

Music therapy is therefore a scientific discipline. It is only a question of establishing a boundary between historical aspects, among which we find legends, and objective research concerning the effect of music and sound on human beings, animals and plants.

History was imbued with magic, omnipotence and suggestion and this is a reason for great interest in theoretical research on music therapy.

Scientific research, on the other hand, will make possible a clear use of the applications of sound and music in the therapeutic field.

We find in the Bible an example of the historical aspect:

"...And so, every time the evil spirit coming from God invested Saul, David took the zither and started to play; Saul calmed down and was better off, because the evil spirit withdrew

from him."

We find, instead, an example of the scientific aspect in Fèrè de la Salpetrière, French physiologist, who studied the influence of music on the working capacity of man with the help of the ergograph of Mosso. He noted that it was above all rhythmic stimuli that contributed to the increase in body performance. He also noted the stimulating influence of music, regardless of rhythm, when intensity was related to tonality: the stimulating effect was more intense in the major tonality than in the minor.3

CHAPTER 6

MUSIC THERAPY: COMPLEX SOUND - HUMAN BEING

This complex consists of:

-elements capable of producing sound stimuli such as: nature, the human body, musical instruments, electronic devices, etc.;

-stimuli such as silence, internal body sounds (heartbeats, joints, intestinal noises, etc.), musical, rhythmic, melodic and harmonic sounds, movements, noises, ultrasounds, infrasounds, words;

-the routes of propagation of vibrations with their physical laws;

-the organs that receive these stimuli, such as the auditory system, internal perception, touch and sight;

-the impression and reception by the nervous system and its relationship with the endocrine, parasympathetic, etc.;

-the psychobiological reaction and the elaboration of the response;

-the response that can be behavioral, motor, sensory, organic, communication through the cry, tears, singing, dancing, music.

Music therapy collaborates with medicine in order to promote the inclusion of the patient in society and the prevention of diseases, both physical and mental.

In music therapy, movement and sound are the same thing or, to be more precise, complete each other.

In each movement a sound is implicit, and each sound generates and is generated by a movement.

Speaking of the regressive effects of sound and music, they are not referred to as the only therapeutic objective: there are sounds capable of producing, in some individuals, totally opposite effects.

One of the deepest phenomena, produced by sound and music, is the ability to cause regressive states in the human being which, for example, is fundamental in the psychiatric application of music therapy.

In the case of developmental disorders, alterations or regressive movements (regression) are recorded in it, which lead back to earlier stages experienced with, more or less, success: oral stage, anal stage or foetal stage.

In other words, in an individual who experiences frustration, there is always a tendency to regret past periods of his life, in which the same experiences were more gratifying, and earlier stages in which the satisfaction was total: the regression is, therefore, a mechanism of defense of the Ego.

In this regard, it is appropriate to insert two conceptual terms: that of "regressive, regenerative sounds" and that of "non-verbal complex".

The former have as their main characteristic the fact that they cause regressive effects in human beings to a greater extent than any other sound, and in a more or less constant way, regardless of the pathology or individual characters. The most common example of regressive sound is the heartbeat.

A "non-verbal complex", on the other hand, means the set of sound and musical elements, movements and acoustic phenomena that cause regressive effects.

It should be pointed out, first of all, that it is possible to open communication channels not only thanks to the production of regressive effects but also according to other characteristics of the musical sound stimuli that are part of the therapeutic process.

Often ergotherapy, phono-audiology, psychotherapy, use in their approach to the patient, communication channels opened by music therapy.

In other cases, the channels of communication do not represent new ways of access to psychic dynamics but only the restructuring of existing ways.

In this process, music therapy often occupies the first ring, since it is used as the first technique of approach, for example in work with autistic children.

Sometimes music therapy is a form of help throughout the process, as in the case where the objective is to obtain compensatory movements in motor rehabilitation or in the release of obsessive structures in deep psychotherapies. After having traced a general profile on music therapy, it seems significant to me to report the comparison that Volterra (1994) made between the function of the musical interpreter and that of the analyst. Both, he maintains, "penetrate a given possibility, modify it without altering it, give another voice to the material constituted influencing its expressiveness".

The listener and the patient reflect themselves and find themselves in this world of sounds and words.

Both find themselves within a different material reorganized according to a precise project, according

144

to a defined line of meanings: in this way, they can glimpse and express interior perspectives that are not known.

In this sense, music and words reveal and structure internal contents. Extending this reflection to the music therapist we can say that its function is, in the first instance, to give voice to the musicality of the patient to facilitate its expression.

In order to carry out this process, the music therapist acts as an interpreter in front of a score, in this case a score made up of the subject and his sonic/musical identity (this manifests itself primarily at the tonic, motor and vocal level); the music therapist also "penetrates" an expressive "possibility" emerging from this material and without transforming the modification in the sense of enhancing it from an aesthetic, communicative and relational point of view; this process is expressed in what is commonly called a sound/musical dialogue, but can also be achieved through specific proposals for listening.

In such contexts the music therapist selects from the material produced by the patient, or from the peculiar way of being of these (from his phenomenal reality), the most significant aspects from a musical, expressive and relational point of view in order to

145

interpret them, structure them musically and communicate them (through an instrumental performance or a listening proposal); the patient can feel understood and contained with respect to his own inner world, and at the same time, urged to express himself in relation to the transmitted models.

The music therapist is therefore an "interpreter" of the expressive potential of the patient, of the signs and meanings that emerge from his body and from his being in the world; he tries with respect to them a maieutic action; the postulate that underlies this intervention provides that the formalized expression of his inner world possesses therapeutic potential. The treatment can continue trying to implement an evolution if not an elaboration of the communicative and relational modalities of the patient, when these require it).

This process presupposes an awareness of the defensive modalities and of the characteristic peculiarities. These aspects can be amplified and highlighted, during the course of the intervention, through specific sound/musical proposals.

The music can also be used as a potential model of change with respect to the personological aspects that characterize the patient.

It is evident, however, that the implementation of such a process necessarily requires access to a phase of verbalization where to focus and process the experiences that emerged during the treatment.

This phase presupposes, like the previous one, having defined and understood the meaning and the meanings (explicit, potential or latent) of the sounds and/or music produced in the music therapy "setting", with respect to the specificity of the patient/musical therapist relationship and the individual specificities.

It is therefore necessary to analyze first of all the ways of interpretation with sound and with music according to the degree of intra and extrapsychic development achieved.

Durif Varembont in 1986 states in this regard that the sound acquires different values and meanings depending on whether the subject is in the psychopathological field of neurosis and psychosis. In neuroses (psychogenic diseases in which the symptoms are the symbolic expression of a psychic conflict that has its roots in the childish history of the subject and is a compromise between desire and defense) the sound acquires its own meaning and becomes a sort of small music of the subject, in a sense comes to take the place of the lost object, the mother, and becomes the image through the game of metaphorical and metonymic substitutions.

The sound, in fact, does not belong only to the real but acquires symbolic values capable of remembering who is absent. In this way it becomes music because it is able to evoke "something"; in this sense it represents the nostalgic attempt to find the lost object forever.

For Varembont, music has this evocative potential only among those subjects who have faced the Oedipal conflict.

It is this level of maturity that allows the aesthetic gratification experienced while listening to a musical work or in artistic creation. It is a relationship with the sound element totally different from the fusional and autoerotic one that the psychotic establishes for example by hitting on a drum with stereotype mode.

In psychoses (psychogenic affections in which we often see them appearing alongside each other criteria such as the inability to adapt socially, the seriousness of the symptoms more or less great, the disruption of the difficulty of communication, the lack of awareness of the morbid state, the loss of contact with reality, the unintelligible character of the disorders, the organic or psychogenetic determinism, the more or

148

less profound and irreversible alterations of the ego), in fact, as in the newborn, there is only the real that resists changing into signifier.

The other is not separated from the Self and does not have a symbolic representation.

The sound element constitutes an event of the real and not of the symbolic, it belongs to the body and does not refer to the image of the body, because, the voice-sound, the voice-body is not yet separated from the voice-language. What is heard is not yet the sign of an absent presence, which could solicit in the child a cry of appeal (e.g. for the mother who hears, without seeing, in the next room).

The sound only evokes the immediacy of a "noise" that addresses no one and represents nothing.

It is a fusional sound, because the Self and the Not Self are not yet differentiated, the sounds of verbal language, the noises, the cries of the newborn are still confused with each other, in particular the voice and the noises of the mother and those of the newborn (in this regard it is better to speak of "Mother voice" and "Voice-child", as proposed by Prof. Lacas, because it is not yet the voice of someone).

The passage from the mother voice to the voice of the mother and therefore to the voice of the child as a subject indicates the progressive separation of the various sounds that are inscribed in a certain musicality and are organized to acquire meaning.

The notes detach themselves from the phonemic noises to function in the order of the articulated signifier. Thus we pass from "sound-noise to sound-music".

By extrapolating these concepts and applying them to the music therapy setting, it emerges that, in relation to the level of evolution of the clinical picture, the meaning of the sounds produced by the patient and the sense attributed by them to the sounds of the operator can present fundamental differences, as well as the relational model that will be defined.

In subjects with prevailing psychotic aspects, the experience of sound will probably be lived with fusional modalities, it will constitute the re-edition of a symbiotic relationship and it will reinforce the autoerotic and narcissistic components of the subject.

Therapist and patient will gratify each other, the first by contrasting the pleasure felt by the other in the relationship with the sound/musical element, the second simply contrasting their own.

It is easy, therefore, that we do not have a real exchange, but only the participation in a fusional experience.

With the term "fusion", used in a different way or, often, as a synonym of symbiosis, is indicated the fantasy of being one with the mother.

This is clear when, in contact with the other, anxieties of fragmentation/dissolution do not emerge, evoked by the perspective of a close relationship.

In other cases, seriously unevolved or regressed on the level of the object relation, the sound/musical element can acquire the characteristics of an autistic object aimed at self-stimulation and at the protection of one's weak Self.

In subjects in which the process of delimitation of the Self with respect to the not Self has been initiated, the musical sound element can acquire other values.

One can observe situations in which the sound becomes a substitute object that, in an almost concrete way, replaces the absent object; cases in which the sound and the music instead acquire greater symbolic peculiarities. The sound then becomes a transitional phenomenon with which to try to recover an original unit; the sounds produced or heard return the presence of the absent mother in a much more vivid way than its image memory.

In more evolved situations the music can be configured as an intermediary instrument, it can become in the relationship with the therapist an instrument of relational mediation and appear to the subject as one between two that for its characteristics of neutrality can facilitate a communicative and relational process.

"... a communication tool able to act therapeutically on the patient within the relationship without creating states of intense alarm ..." the elements that characterize it are the real existence, the harmlessness, the malleability; also allows communication, replacing the bond and keeping it at a distance, is adaptable to the needs of the subject, is identifiable.

Dr. Pennec, head of the music therapy service of the hospital Sud La Roche sur Yon, believes that often within a music therapy relationship the music represents the request for a relationship with a therapist and not with a music therapist.

Music therefore acts as a counterphobic object that allows the patient to face a therapeutic relationship, otherwise distressing and unsustainable.

Music is also linked to the patient's experience and can be included in a system of parental references.

In the music therapy relationship, "three subjects" are thus organized, to whom a role can be attributed: the role of the child, which is often attributed to the patient, that of music-father, music-mother and that of therapist-mother and therapist-father.

In a later evolutionary stage music can lose its value as a counterphobic object, mediator of the relationship, and become the "container" of the music therapy relationship.

In other cases, finally, narcissistic problems can be highlighted.

The musical becomes a sort of magic mirror that refers to the patient an ideal and omnipotent image; the same therapeutic couple can be configured as ideal and aconflictual, reinforced in this by a gratifying and complacent use of the sound/musical element.

AREAS OF INTERVENTION

When we talk about music therapy, the term "music" refers to a set of sound/musical materials not usually included within the concept of "Musical Art". In fact, they can be used in various ways:

-Daily, bodily, unorganized vowel sounds-noises;

-Daily, bodily, organized vowel sounds-noises;

-Infrasound, ultrasound;

-Music understood in a common sense.

In the selection of the sound/musical material we do not refer to aesthetic and/or cultural assumptions (the use of elements commonly appreciated as music) but to clinical and operational assumptions (the use of elements that can have a meaning in the project of intervention).

Any acoustic event that can be perceived and not by the auditory apparatus (but in this case transmitted by tactile-vibratory means) without a pre-established hierarchy of values can be used.

The sound/musical element can acquire music therapy values in two different areas:

PSYCHOTHERAPY AND REHABILITATION.

PSYCHOTHERAPY

In the approach with subjects that are particularly regressed or not evolved in terms of objective relations (infantile psychosis and adult psychosis, infantile cerebropathies), music therapy represents an extra-verbal communication channel that is often able to favour the expression of the patient and the overcoming of situations of isolation, allowing access to a dimension of interpersonal relations.

With regard to a less compromised case study (psychoneurosis, personality disorders, borderline pictures), it can be a welcoming and containing tool that favours the emergence of emotions and subjective experiences and can subsequently act as a model of change in one's own internal world.

REHABILITATION

The gratification derived from the fruition of the sound/musical element can facilitate the activation of a certain function (motor, vocal, etc. ...); at the same time, the

155

formal aspects of the sound/musical sequence used constitute the model within which this function is articulated.

As Postacchini states in 1986, the rehabilitative intervention considered in a perspective of activation, containment and structuring, can be addressed to three main areas of disorder:

Firstly, neurosensory disorders: the deaf child and the blind child;

The second area of intervention concerns neuromotor disorders;

the third area concerns neuropsychological disorders (aphasia, apressia, agnosia).

METHODOLOGICAL ASPECTS

There are two common application modes: active music therapy and receptive music therapy.

Active music therapy is defined as the direct manipulation of a musical instrument (or common everyday objects used with sound/musical modalities). The instrumentarium is mostly made up of the musical material of the Orff methodology: these are musical instruments characterized by easy manipulation, even in the absence of a specific musical competence, and by a rich range of timbres and tones.

The diction music therapy receptive refers to a practice of listening to sound/musical differently aimed at the intervention of an intervention program.

This terminology is preferred to that of passive music therapy to overcome the misunderstanding of a pseudopharmacological application of the sound/musical element and to emphasize that even listening should be considered an active process in which the subject recreates and transforms the musical and sound proposal.

The methodological procedure of the music therapy intervention foresees a specific investigation, aimed at determining the sound/musical characteristics of the subject and of the social and family environment of origin, and a preliminary phase of observation and evaluation which will be followed by the elaboration of an operational project.

The information, obtained if possible from interviews with the patient or his family, is collected in special cards, as well as the phase of observation that takes into account: the behavior of the subject in his usual environment, the mode of exploration and manipulation of music therapy instruments, the characteristics of vocal production and speech, the characteristics of body rhythm, the patient's response to listening to a specific sound/musical sequence (used in order to probe its musical receptivity, the response to listening to the re-listening of personal sound/musical productions, the response to relational proposals rhythmic-body and sound/musical implemented by the music therapist.

These aspects analyzed and evaluated on the basis of specific parameters sound/musical and communicative-relational will provide the elements for the development of a project of intervention.

The observation tries to highlight with which strategies the subject faces the proposed experience and the characteristics of its sound/musical production. These aspects are then evaluated in terms of the possible symbolic meaning that they can assume.

It is also essential to know that the listening proposed to subjects with serious cognitive and relational deficits must include a sound/musical sequence characterized by body sounds and rhythms that then evolve into elementary musical structures and always connected to the body dimension of the musical experience.

The proposal to listen to subjects who are normodote can include, in addition to the sequence described above, pieces and extracts of music classified differently in relation to the formal aspects and the prevailing affective tonality.

An in-depth evaluation of the clinical aspects and of the peculiar sound/musical characteristics of the subject must be carried out following the description of the following aspects:

-The basic neuropsychological functional structure related to sensory and motor functioning;

-The type of learning, which may or may not be of a processing type;

-The object relation, of pregenital or genital type, according to the level of mature development;

-Predictable complications, related to the type of expression (Postacchini 1994).

The "neuropsychological functional structure" is characterized by the level of functioning of the sensory and motor analyzers, that is, by a dynamic description of the analyzer that involves a high degree of dynamic balance and fluidity of the passages between moments in which accumulations of sensory and perceptual elements prevail (see, feel, act, touch = BETA elements) and moments in which a process of mental elaboration is initiated (see, listen, discriminate, perform = ALFA elements), with moments of possible harmony, sensory or mental between the various analyzers and moments in which some operate in the mental and others in the sensory resulting in a situation of disharmony.

The "types of learning" described by G.Moretti are characterized by the following levels:

Situations in which the stimulus is massively decoded and the response is massively provided

Ontogenetically it is represented by the reflected activities susceptible to conditioned learning.

Situations in which the stimulus can be decoded for a generic character and the response coded according to similar strategies.

Ontogenetically, it is the response of the child's smile to the presentation of the maternal face; and also the response to situations of danger or palatability on the part of a brain-damaged person.

The learning will be at selective range, with a possible training capacity even if reduced, there are the concepts of space, time and speed.

Situations in which the stimulus can be decoded, and the response be encoded within a category. Ontogenetically it corresponds to the child's discrimination between the mother and the outside world.

The dynamics of the process in this case is linguistically determined; learning occurs by symbolisation and will be reversible.

Situations in which the stimulus is decoded and the response encoded by modalization.

Ontogenetically it corresponds to the maturation of the fifteenth month: at this level it is possible to recognize the abstract characters of a stimulus; learning will be symbolic, subject to selective inhibition, influenced by values and self-determined. This is the normal learning level.

The "object relation" includes:

an archaic, pregenital situation, characterized by a scarce capacity for symbolizing and deferring tensions, lability of attention and containment of aggression; a recognition of the partial object, that is, in a confusing way for those properties that are functional to the needs of the child and not for the characteristics that are its own.

161

Or, a more mature situation, of the genital type, characterized by a total recognition of the object, i.e. evaluated as such, with the properties that compete with it and the feelings that characterize it, not in function of the needs of the child, but of the real cognitive and emotional conditions in which the object is found. In this sense, the relationship will be mature; non-confusive, and capable of distinguishing differences and similarities.

The type of predictable complications depends directly on the type of "prevention" implemented:
primary: is the prevention of the causes of the disease. In the case of mental or neurological diseases, primary prevention still remains a utopian attitude because the causes are not always known;
secondary: prevention of the complications of an already stabilised deficit. About the causes of a disease
mental, we can imagine that for a schizophrenic, stabilizing his conduct, his behavior, his communicative styles, can be a good way to promote a degree of social inclusion;
tertiary: to intervene by stabilizing the complications where they have already occurred. In serious

schizophrenic pathologies, with autistic closures, we can imagine that talking with that patient, inside his autistic shell, is the only possible way of stabilization.

PRINCIPLES OF MUSIC THERAPY

Music therapy, as a methodology and technique of clinical application, is based on two principles:
the ISO principle,
the intermediate object.

These two principles are not the exclusive prerogative of music therapy, since they can be the basis of many other non-verbal techniques. However, in music therapy, they take on particular characteristics.
ISO principle

Altshuler, in his clinical observations on the application of music therapy, observed that depressed people respond better to stimulation produced by means of sad and melancholic music, rather than cheerful music.

163

"Neurotic subjects, whose mental time is faster, respond better to a cheerful person than to a andante.

On the basis of these observations, the concept of "iso" was elaborated little by little as a fundamental principle of music therapy, both on a theoretical and practical level.

Iso means "equal" and synthesizes the notion of the existence of a sound or a set of sounds or internal sound phenomena that characterize and individualize us. It is a sound phenomenon and internal movement that summarizes our sound archetypes, our intrauterine sound experience and our sound experience of birth, childhood and our present age.

It is a sound structured within a sound mosaic which is structured, in turn, with time and which is, fundamentally, in perpetual movement.

To generate a channel of communication between therapist and patient, the mental time of the patient must coincide with the musical sound time performed by the music therapist: this could, however, suggest an iso too intellectual and rigid, measured with the parameters of intensity, timbre, height, etc..

In fact, the iso is a dynamic element that potentially has in itself all the strength of present and past perception.

For this reason, in the therapeutic context, the communication channel is really open when it is possible to discover the patient's iso through the coincidence of that of the therapist.

We can distinguish between a Gestaltic ISO, a Complementary ISO, a Group ISO and a Universal ISO.

The Gestaltic ISO is the dynamic mosaic that characterizes the individual, the iso that allows us to discover what is the channel of communication par excellence of the subject with whom we try to establish a therapeutic relationship.

By this we mean the concept of Gestalt in the sense in which it was originally understood by Wertheimer,

"The psychology of Gestalt highlights the need to return to the original perception, to immediate experience, not altered by a preconceived hypothesis that deforms the reality of the phenomenon observed.

It follows that perception does not grasp a set of elements, but a whole".

The subject does not perceive a set of elementary sounds, but a global sensation.

The Complementary ISO is the set of those small changes that take place every day or in every music therapy session under the effect of environmental and dynamic circumstances; it represents, that is, the momentary fluctuation of the gestalt iso under the effect of specific environmental circumstances.

The Group ISO is intimately connected to the social scheme within which the individual evolves. It takes a certain amount of time for the group iso to establish and structure itself: it will often depend on the good composition of the group and on the music therapist's knowledge of each patient's individual iso.

The group iso is fundamental to reach a unity of integration in a therapeutic group in a non-verbal context; it is a dynamic that pervades the group as the synthesis itself of all sound identities.

M.E. Grebe, in his article "Cultural aspects of music therapy: relations between anthropology, ethnomusicology and music therapy". takes up the concept of group iso and states that it is "the sound identity of a human group, as a product of the latent musical affinities developed in each of its members".

Given its characteristics, the notion of group iso leads directly to the concept of ethnic identity. A nation or people of complex culture brings together in itself a heterogeneous set of cultural, sub-cultural, or cultural minorities; that is, cultural parts of a whole.

Although these groups are different from region to region, they are essentially distinguished by biological (race), cultural (language), geographical (regions) signs, each of which gives the individual members an ethnic identity or affective self-identification with the other members of the group and, consequently, through relatively frequent hostility towards strangers to the group.

Consequently, ethnic cultural identity cannot be separated from sound identity (iso) and depends both on the dynamic learning processes of one's own culture and on the stability or change of cultural rules. However, it is considered fundamental to affirm that to the group iso it is necessary to add, in order to fully understand it, the idiosyncrasy or the set of idiosyncrasies of the individual members of the given group; this expands what M. E. Grebe maintains in the sense that the iso depends on the history of gestation and on the infantile history of the individual.

CHAPTER 7

HAPPY: HOW TO GET OUT OF THE DCA TUNNEL

"Happiness is born of loneliness as a flower from the earth. Relationships with others are the rain that nourishes the earth. To seek happiness while avoiding loneliness is like watering the bare rock, hoping that flowers will be born there".

The most important ethical commitment is to be happy in the now, moment by moment, happy with what is there, as it is.

An unhappy person is basically a person prey to his Ego. As such, he does not love anyone, but feeds on contempt, starting with contempt for himself.

Love your neighbor as yourself becomes possible only if you are happy inside, that is, if you are free from the domain of the Ego.

Happiness, unlike what is commonly thought, is not the result of the circumstances of life, more or less favorable. Rather, it arises naturally from the daily practice of the qualities of being, such as appreciation, gratitude, generosity, integrity, compassion.

Those who are happy emanate positive waves that are good for all people around. And, given the nature of being together, doing good to others is doing good to oneself.

In turn, unhappiness originates from the practice of mental pollutants, such as anger, resentment, ingratitude, contempt, envy, suspicion, repression. Pollutants are the means that the Ego uses to increase its power over the person. Naturally, in order to pursue this strategy, he must make it completely unconscious: the person must not even have the suspicion that he is committing himself with all his heart to pursue his own evil. On the contrary, he must believe that he is making the right moves to "defend himself", "protect himself", "pursue his own interests". That is why the fundamental characteristic of the Ego is the distortion of reality, or, in simple terms, the systematic lie. Lies are necessary to keep the person in ignorance. But the individual Ego cannot do everything on its own. It would not be able to do so. The individual ego is built through the internalization of the collective ego. That is why it is so important, in order to melt one's neurosis, to begin to become aware of its cultural and collective determinants.

From a physical point of view, unhappiness is a train of negative waves, which produces malaise or illness. It's a clamorous music, which hurts the ear and the heart. Like a train of waves, unhappiness spreads to the surrounding environment, contaminating the people around unless they have developed sufficient awareness to escape the phenomenon of resonance. The presence of an unhappy person can make a group depressed. Everyone feels less well, and to avoid this displeasure, they easily make counter-productive moves (see below).

Those who are happy are an example that it is desirable to follow. Of course there may be those who see in the happiness of others a threat: a threat to their own power to impose their own bad mood and through that condition relatives, friends, acquaintances. In other words, leaders rooted in the qualities of being are poorly seen by negative selfish leaders.

HAPPY PARENTS HAVE MUCH MORE POWER TO EDUCATE THEIR CHILDREN.

The happy means that they value happiness. Happy parents value what can bring happiness to their children: affection, presence, empathy, love. They do not therefore need to compensate them for their shortcomings, to spoil them, to give in to blackmail. Moreover, the children see in the parents models of how they themselves can become in the future by following their example. If the parents are sad and in a bad mood, the children will not want to follow them. If they try to teach them something, they will lack leadership. The children will oppose: I don't want to become like you!

The less evolved internal parts, the sub-personalities, behave like their children: they have no intention of following the directives of an unhappy i-government! They will reject his leadership. They will oppose and continue to do so on their own terms. But being very small as a mental age, their contribution will be scarcely appreciable, if not even harmful or devastating. All these things will feed the unhappiness of the poor i-government, less and less able to govern and more and more ready to complain and suffer.

In our philosophy, happiness has often been confused with pleasure, without looking at the consequences that different types of pleasure bring with them.

Some pleasures are actually full of poison, and obscure the possibility of being happy.

If a wound itches me, scratching me offers a momentary pleasure. But if I keep scratching, what will happen? If I feel down, I look for relief in alcohol or food. But in the long run, where does this choice take me?

In the Buddhist view, happiness means joy of being, without causes, without conditions. Sukha, ananda, do not depend on performance, appearance, success, health, even if they can be influenced by it.

From our point of view, bad mood is one of the most subtle forms of racketeering, that is, psychological mafia, through which one person steals energy from another, without becoming happy.

In other words, it is an aggressive equivalent, a passive-aggressive form: it hurts by concealing its destructive nature. Since it is a widespread form, it is easy for those who practice it to avoid feedback and confrontation. In this way it can continue on this path for years, without having the slightest awareness of it, and sowing around many seeds of unhappiness.

The Ego, which feeds on unhappiness, finds in this form a simple and effective way to increase its power over the person, the couple, the family, the group where it can exercise it.

People around, especially those predisposed to suffer from guilt, those who believe that the happiness of others depends on their behavior, thus fall into a trap very risky: to escape the burden of bad mood of a partner or friend, begin to investigate his unmet needs, getting in response a sequence of complaints: I miss this, I need that, there is this terrible thing that I can not eliminate etc.. At this point they feel obliged to soothe the pain of the other, starting to act on his behalf or making promises that will often require a much greater commitment than expected, given the passivity of the person suffering.

Every promise becomes debt. And now the relationship with the other, whining or in a bad mood, becomes a sort of work that becomes increasingly heavy. From a fraternal relationship, of help, it becomes a parasitic relationship, in which one of the two continues to give, and the other to receive and disperse in the wind. Before there was one unhappy person, now there are two. The Ego of both can celebrate. Helping the other never means doing things in his place, taking on his loads, assuming his commitments and responsibilities. This only weakens the other, making him more and more succulent and fuelling his anger and resentment. That is precisely those pollutants that prevent him from seeing reality as it is, in its infinite possibilities.

The aid is such only if it is accompanied by all the qualities of being. Love, in the first place. And loving a person means fostering his evolution, his psychological and spiritual growth. That is to say, to favour the development of one's resources and of an interior government inspired by the messages of the soul, rather than by the propaganda of the Ego. Here lies the difference between piety and compassion. Pity sees in the other only its problems. Compassion, in addition to problems, sees its strength and resources. It sees in the problems only symptoms of the distorted way of observing the world. Pity makes us replace the other: you are a poor man, I am superior, in conditions much better than yours. Compassion sees in the pain of the other a reflection of his own pain: I, on a deep level, am like you, a stream that floats in the great river of life. I have my limits, as you have yours. But I know that there is something greater that can help us both: the growth of awareness and the openness of heart.

When the heart is closed, the eyes don't really see reality, but they invent it on a healthy basis. The map that guides our lives is therefore deeply false and distorted. It is a paranoid map, which sees obstacles and enemies everywhere.

Helping a person basically means this: encouraging the opening of his heart through the opening of his own presence and awareness.

The first step in this direction is to free oneself from feelings of guilt, inadequacy, unworthiness. All radical neurotics that depend on the practice of judgement, criticism, and dutifulness, through which the oppressive and selfish culture weakens its members, making them slaves to false perceptions and induced needs, certainly incapable of a revolution that goes to the center of the problems: unmasking the impersonal and perverse nature of the Ego and power domination.

DCA CARE WITH MUSIC THERAPY

Successful treatment depends on timely diagnosis and treatment, usually by a team of specialists. The staff includes, among others, psychiatrists, psychologists and nutritionists to whom it is possible to add, as a valid support, a music therapy path that aims to open sensory and emotional channels through which the person can re-enter into contact with their body, the emotional experiences that involve it and the behaviors that result, reflecting on the image that they have of themselves and on the way to relate to each other by themselves.

In the absence of a willingness to communicate and share verbally the internal emotional states, music therapy is a valuable aid that, starting from a "communication without words" of feelings and emotions, gradually leads the subject in the field of memories, feelings, blocks never overcome, which may emerge spontaneously after a listening or a real musical performance. Only in this way will it be easier to access the experience of the person and solve those knots, perhaps present for some time, that have generated so much suffering. In this way, a sort of "bridge" will be built between the internal and external worlds, creating a path through which to pass from the possibility of expressing one's own emotions to the ability to decode and regulate them. We know in fact that our emotions are in constant flow and always changeable: but when one of them begins to impose itself on the others and to dominate our psyche, it can cause an imbalance that it is opportune to correct by going to identify, make emerge and resolve the founding cause that has generated such imbalance.

But the ability to live, feel, express and control emotions is a quality that not everyone possesses in equal measure and that, in some circumstances, it may be useful to enhance or acquire totally. In 1990, this ability was defined by Peter Salovey and John D. Mayer as "emotional intelligence": it allows the awareness of one's own emotional experiences and control over their expression, as well as the ability to tolerate frustration, to recognize the emotional states of others (empathy) and, on the basis of the same, to manage social relationships. In this context, music therapy, through the use of the sound-musical parameter, invites the person to the use of different sensory channels, perceptual and expressive that tend to the symbolic communication of emotions and the sharing of them, giving rise to a creative process that has in itself a significant value cathartic and therapeutic.